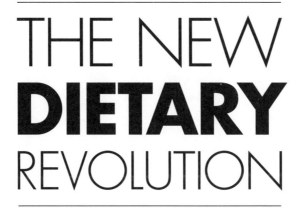

THE NEW
DIETARY
REVOLUTION

Distribution Codirect Inc.
4335, Verdun Street
Verdun Qc
H4G 1L6
(514) 767-1745 / 1 800 268-1007

© 1999, Distribution Codirect Inc.

ISBN : 0-9730502-0-9

Cover : Bernard Langlois
Graphic design : Composition Monika, Québec

PRINTED IN CANADA

THE NEW
DIETARY
REVOLUTION

Dr MAURICE LAROCQUE
with the collaboration of Dr Harry J. Lefebre

Summary

Introduction   How Does It Work?   13

PART ONE

The New Dietary Revolution

Chapter 1   A New Discovery: Sugar Can Be as
Hazardous as Fat   17

The Experts Are Wrong.   17

The Real Culprit: Hyperinsulinemia . .   17

It's Not a Question of Willpower.   18

Will Nutrition Undergo Major
Changes?   19

In the Middle of a Revolution.   20

A Few Objections   21

The New Recommendations.   22

In Conclusion   23

Chapter 2   For a Better Understanding   25

Different Types of Carbohydrates   25

Glycemic Index.   26

Insulin Kills   27

Mechanism of Action   28

Metabolic Syndrome.   29

Hypoglycemia.   30

Sugar Substitutes   30

Chapter 3   Personalized Method   33

Your Caloric Requirements   33

Your Protein Requirements.   34

Your Carbohydrate Requirements. . . .   35

Your Fat Requirements   36

Chapter 4   Tips for Motivation and Good Health.   39

Setting Success Goals   39

The Dimmer Switch   41

Preventing and Coping with a Lapse .   43

The Scale.   45

Calorie Banking   47

Realistic Goals.   48

Successful Restarting Starts with
Decreasing Guilt   50

"Treat" vs "Cheat"   51

Triple "A" Process for Positive Change.   52

Taking Care of "Numero Uno"   54

Diet Saboteurs   57

"Toughest Challenge of One's Life" . .   59

PART TWO

The Recipes

Recipes that will satisfy your hunger.   61

Index.   291

Acknowledgements

We would like to thank the following people for their invaluable help:

Johanne Vachon, Director of the Maurice Larocque and Associates clinics (1490 Sherbrooke West, Montreal H3G 1L3 and 4335 Verdun, Verdun H4G 1L6) and Murielle Chauviteau, Administrative Assistant for Maurice Larocque and Associates.

In particular, we would also like to thank Andrea Rubin, McGill nutrition student, for her excellent recipes.

About the authors

Maurice Larocque, MD, has practiced medicine since 1970 and has been especially active in the treatment of obesity for over 25 years. He is the inventor of MENTAL WEIGHT, a revolutionary concept for treating obesity. He is also the author of seven books (including the best sellers *Be Thin Through Motivation, Be Thin and Self-Confident, Be Thin Master Your Emotions, Be Thin Day by Day*) and fifteen self-help audio-cassettes on effective mind-programming techniques. He is recognized internationally in his field. He is often asked to present the results of his many studies at different conferences throughout the world. Considered a leader by his peers, Dr. Larocque is a member of the New York Academy of Science, American Sports Medicine Association, American Society of Bariatric Physicians (ASBP) and the North American Association for the Study of Obesity (NAASO). Since 1982, he has been president of the Bariatric Physicians Association (AMTO).

Harry J. Lefebre, MD, has been a member of the Alberta College of Physicians and Surgeons since 1974. Dr. Lefebre was a family doctor up until he limited his medical practice to Bariatrics in 1985. He is diplomate of the American Board of Bariatric Medicine (ABBM). He has been a member of the American Society of Bariatric Physicians (ASBP) since 1983 and was their trustee in 2001. He has also been an associate member of the North American Association for Study of Obesity (NAASO) since 1993. Highly active in his community, fighting obesity is his main concern.

Dr. Lefebre and Dr. Larocque joined forces in the eighties.

How Does It Work?

In the area of nutrition, weight loss or health, hardly a week goes by without new information or advertising contradicting what was previously said. Who is telling the truth?

As more and more people are becoming aware of the importance of a good diet to remain slim and healthy, a wide variety of con artists are more than happy to extol the values of their miracle product, food or method. Money is the motivator for these charlatans and justifies all their lies. It seems that the bigger the lie, the more chance it will be believed. Most people who are suffering from obesity or poor health would do anything to change their situation and therefore are potentially easy victims.

Even more disturbing are the often contradictory messages of scientists, doctors or healthcare professionals. Everyone has his own sure-fire recipe! In fact, the official message of the authorities develops and changes quickly. For example, not so long ago, they recommended using margarine to prevent heart disease; we were advised not to use butter and other fats. We now know that hydrogenated margarine is as much, if not more, hazardous for your health as butter.

In fact, we are right in the middle of a new diet revolution. The new target: sugar, even that found in bread or pasta (which are considered healthy). The latest studies lead us to believe that it is even worse for our health than fat.

However, the official authorities on nutrition have always stated that with a well-balanced diet, there's no need to take food supplements. However, recent studies, especially those on antioxidants, show the opposite.

So, who is telling the truth? Well... you can believe whomever you want. However, you should know that the information in this book comes from thirty years of experience in the field of nutrition and weight loss and are based on the most recent discoveries (which shatter our past beliefs).

The thousands of testimonies that we received led us to write this book so that we can share with a great number of people the principles of a healthy diet, which is a measurement of good health. The tips in this book will help you substantially reduce the risk of heart disease, diabetes and cancer. You will see that prevention tastes good! These recipes will allow you to enjoy your food without feeling unbearably hungry.

The most extraordinary thing is that the recommendations – and there are only four of them – are easy to incorporate into your new lifestyle and are extremely effective. Yes! You read that correctly, there are only four tips to being slim and healthy. What's more, our recipes respect all dietary criteria of the new scientific standards that we are recommending.

Enjoy the book and the meals in good health!

PART ONE

The
New Dietary
Revolution

Chapter 1

A New Discovery:
Sugar Can Be as Hazardous as Fat*

In February 1998, I wrote the following in the Health Motivation newsletter:

The Experts Are Wrong

The current creed of the nutrition authorities is to promote a high-carbohydrate diet (slow assimilation sugars), primarily found in bread and whole-grain cereals, fruits, vegetables and legumes.

This position taken by the scientists is based on the results of their studies, which identified fat, especially animal fat, as being the main factor responsible for many health problems, including heart disease. Nowadays, since our sources of protein are often rich in fat (for example, beef), this led them to immediately jump to conclusions and recommend lowering the consumption of meat. I call that throwing the baby out with the bathwater. Since you have to eat *something*, they recommended increasing the amount of carbohydrates, which, once digested, become sugar in the blood.

The Real Culprit: Hyperinsulinemia

Experience has shown that a very high number of people who follow a high-carbohydrate diet are often hungry a few hours

---

after eating. They lack energy and find it difficult to lose and maintain weight. The most recent discoveries have allowed us to identify an additional surplus of insulin in the blood, which is primarily responsible for the excess weight. A recent American study, published in 1997, confirms this observation. Consumption of carbohydrates by people in good health (whose parents are diabetic) acutely stimulates the production of insulin, which, in turn, stimulates appetite (this mechanism is yet unknown and not necessarily linked to hypoglycemia) and leads to weight gain.

It's Not a Question of Willpower

We also know that proteins are the most effective food for decreasing appetite and creating a feeling of fullness for at least four hours. If you suffer from being overweight, sugar cravings, fatigue or mood swings that you can't explain, or if you have a family history of diabetes, you must absolutely avoid eating refined sugar, and eat smaller portions of carbohydrates along with a source of protein. So it's not your willpower that's at fault; it's your metabolism.

Here are a few general tips to make sure you are eating well:

- Eat at least **three meals** a day with a **maximum of four hours between each of them.** Some people who are very sensitive to sugar may need to eat every three hours;

- With **each meal**, have a source of **protein** (very lean meat, fish, skinless chicken, egg whites, fat free milk products, legumes or protein supplements);

- Systematically **avoid** eating all **refined sugars**;

- **Pay attention** to your carbohydrate intake (e.g.: bread, pasta, fruits): eat small quantities of them, preferably in conjunction with a source of protein;

- **Eat more dietary fiber.**

There are two types of dietary fiber: soluble and insoluble. Each, in its own way, plays an important role in maintaining good health. Soluble fibers, along with a low-fat diet, help especially to lower the blood cholesterol rate in people suffering from hypercholesterolemia and lower the blood sugar level. Barley, grapefruit, artichokes and oat bran are good sources of this type of fiber, as are psyllium-based laxatives (Metamucil™), fruits, vegetables and legumes.

* * *

And now look at what I wrote a year and a half later reporting on the revelations in December 1998 by Professor Walter Willett from the School of Public Health at Harvard University.

Will Nutrition Undergo Major Changes?

Over the past few years, were our experts wrong about their nutritional advice? It seems that **this may be the case**.

We have been told to cut our fat intake as much as possible in order to prevent heart disease. However, according to the preliminary results of two major American studies, there is a link between **"modern" diseases** and **sugar** consumption. Refined white sugar is found in candy and soft drinks, but also in "good" foods such as **bread** and **pasta**.

For the past twelve years, Professor Walter Willett of Harvard University has headed two studies involving data on 120,000 health professionals. His mission: to discover the nutritional factors that will likely to keep the current epidemic of chronic disease such as, cancer, heart disease, diabetes and obesity under control.

"I believe we have found the answer", he says. "Quickly absorbed sugars such as those found in potatoes, white bread, pasta, rice and refined sugars may be linked to heart disease.

Our findings identify insulin as the culprit. The more resistant a person is to insulin, the more harmful sugar is to him."

By studying the nutritional behavior of 915 diabetics, it appeared that people who ate large amounts of quickly absorbed sugars increased their risk of diabetes by 50 %. These studies also identified a protective effect: the **fiber** found in cereal decreases this risk by 30 %. When a person consumes large amounts of quickly absorbed sugars and little fiber, the risk for diabetes goes up 2.17 times in men and 2.5 times in women.

Other conclusions: fat is not the main reason a person becomes diabetic, nor for the increased risk of colon and breast cancer. A year earlier, Walter Willett summarized his research findings on this topic: "Instead, we have been troubled by what we have found. When fat consumption was very low, the risk of breast cancer increased twofold. This led us question our Western diet, rich in refined carbohydrates."

I fully agree with Professor Willett's conclusions. Over the past 20 years, my experience with thousands of patients confirms his conclusions and reinforces the soundness of our food recommendations during weight loss and maintenance.

What to make of the official recommendations?

I believe the recommendations to eat 6 to 11 portions of bread, cereal, rice and pasta every day are clearly wrong and lead to heart disease and obesity.

But how do carbohydrates lead to obesity? After eating a meal rich in sugars, insulin is activated, causing the blood glucose (sugar) to drop too low, which causes you to consume more sugar, once again leading to a drop in blood sugar.

In addition, insulin is the hormone that puts weight on people.

In the Middle of a Revolution

We are experiencing a bona fide nutritional revolution. According to Professor Willett, "I hear nutritionists who say that you cannot become fat from eating carbohydrates. That's completely absurd. [...] Anyone can become fat by consuming too many calories. And most calories come from carbohydrates, and not from fat. In the United States, people have lowered the amount of fat in their diets, but increased their number of calories, because they are eating more refined carbohydrates. I think that the explosion of cases of obesity in the United States, like in other countries, is due to the fact that people believe that they won't put on weight by eating carbohydrates."

The problem is compounded by the fact that fat has long been held responsible for the increase in diseases such as colon and breast cancers. Nowadays, many epidemiological studies have not been able to prove that the increased risk for these diseases is due to a high-fat diet.

Today, many studies conducted throughout the world have focused on the role of quick-absorbing carbohydrates in our diet and point the finger at insulin for being responsible for our so-called "civilized" diseases, especially for colon cancer.

A Few Objections

Some people have raised some doubts about the conclusions of these Western studies, since, in Asia, people consume large amounts of white rice (a quick-absorbing carbohydrate) and do not suffer from our so-called "civilized" diseases. However, it seems that the Chinese farmers tolerate carbohydrates better because of different factors:

- They eat few calories, are very thin, and often underweight;
- They consume little saturated fats and red meat;
- They are far more physically active and do manual work in the fields;
- They are not resistant to insulin.

In fact, the lifestyle of most Oriental peoples is completely different from people in the West. As Westerners, we definitely have a lot we could learn from their behavior.

The New Recommendations

Here are the recommendations – four simple principles – that I would give based on these new observations:

1. Move more

It is extremely important to do at least a minimum amount of exercise. We now know that even light physical activity helps prevent insulin resistance and hyperinsulinemia, which are responsible for our "civilized" diseases. What is the ideal activity? It's what you like to do and that you want to do often.

For most of us, walking is the easiest and most appropriate activity. I'd advise that you start slowly, and walk at a comfortable pace. A few minutes a day or every two days may be enough to start. When you feel comfortable with this routine, increase it by five minutes each week, until you're walking 45 minutes a day, five days a week at a speed that will make you slightly out of breath.

2. Replace saturated fat

Very recent studies have shown that saturated fats stimulate the secretion of insulin, which, in turn, increases the blood cholesterol levels and the formation of plaque in the arteries. Therefore, it is important to replace saturated fats, especially those of animal origin, such as red meat, cold cuts, chicken skin, non-skim milk products, fats (butter, mayonnaise, vinaigrettes), by mono – and poly – non-saturated fats of vegetable origin. Note that "replace" does not mean you can't eat them at all: reasonable and occasional consumption will not harm you.

As well, try to avoid trans fatty acids, often found in margarines and are made of **hydrogenated** vegetable oil. These fats lead to hardened arteries.

Canola, safflower, corn, sesame, soy, sunflower, linseed and olive oils are excellent. However, be careful about the amount, since all these oils contain as many calories as other fats, that is 45 calories for 5 ml (1 tsp.). In particular, **eat fish, since it protects against heart disease**.

3. Avoid eating quick-absorbing carbohydrates

Many researchers deplore the fact that industries modify their foods using all sorts of techniques, including refining. This increases the rate at which carbohydrate is absorbed, and reduces or even eliminates their vitamin, natural mineral salts and fiber content.

Therefore, stay away from refined sugar, sweets, soft drinks and jams. Pay attention to the type of carbohydrates that you eat. Choose the ones that are absorbed slowly. White bread, white rice, potatoes and pasta are all quick-absorbing carbohydrates that stimulate insulin production and therefore must be eaten very moderately.

Always choose food rich in fiber (as unrefined as possible).

An important tip: always eat quick-absorbing sugars with a source of protein or at the end of the meal. Their absorption will thus be slowed down, minimizing the secretion of insulin.

4. Eat some protein every four hours

Proteins, which are the most effective nutrient for creating a feeling of fullness, cut appetite for at least four hours in most people. Moreover, they hardly stimulate insulin secretion. Studies have shown that when we eat proteins, spontaneously our appetite decreases, which means we eat fewer calories. The best sources of protein are fish, lentils and lean white meat. If you eat red meat, remove all visible fat.

For most women, it is enough to eat the equivalent of 120 g (4 oz) meat (uncooked weight) with each meal. For men this number goes up to 150 g (5 oz). Skim milk products are also good sources of protein.

In conclusion

Recent discoveries confirm the importance of physical activity, a balanced diet and a healthy weight. Move more, eat less, avoid saturated fats and sugar, and eat protein every four hours. If you follow these recommendations, I promise that you will no longer have any sugar cravings; and, more importantly, you will be able to reach and maintain your healthy weight.

Chapter 2

For a Better Understanding

Different Types of Carbohydrates

Carbohydrates are found, for example, in pasta and all sugars. There are two types of carbohydrates: quick absorption carbohydrates and slow absorption carbohydrates. They are the body's main sources of energy. When we differentiate them based on their chemical structure, carbohydrates can be referred to as:

- **simple:**
- – glucose (refined sugar),
- – fructose (fruit sugar);
- **complex:**
- – saccharose (beet sugar or sugarcane),
- – lactose (milk sugar),
- – maltose (sugar transformed from starch).

Plants, through the sun's energy, synthesize carbohydrates (in particular glucose, fructose and saccharose). Depending on the type of fruit, the quantities of these different sugars vary, as well as their mode and rate of absorption, which explains why they have a different glycemic index.

Seeds, tubers and roots convert carbohydrates into starch. Cereals, potatoes and sweet corn are especially high in starch.

Their transformation through grinding and cooking increases their digestibility.

The cellular walls of plants also contain carbohydrates, but their structure makes them very stable and difficult to digest. These carbohydrates are dietary fiber, which slows down the passage of glucose into the blood while speeding up the abdominal transit. Below are the reasons why they prevent constipation.

Glycemic Index

The glycemic index (GI) – a popular term at the moment – is a physiological measurement that evaluates the rate of absorption of sugars found in food. To measure it, nutrition specialists give a person food containing 50 g (nearly 2 oz) of carbohydrates, and then measure the blood glucose levels every 30 minutes for three hours. Then they compare the curve with that of a reference food: white bread. The lower the glycemic index, the slower the absorption of the sugar into the blood; on the contrary, the higher the glycemic index, the faster the absorption of the sugar and the higher the insulin secreted.

Fiber-rich food has a relatively lower GI, whereas refined food has a high GI. During a meal, the GI of a food is **changed** depending on which **food** is eaten **along with it**. For example, pasta GI is lower with meat sauce.

White sugar is made up of equal parts of glucose and fructose. Fructose influences blood sugar levels far less than glucose, which has a lower GI than we would think.

The glycemic index of some food

High GI: > 70 Moderate GI: between 40 and 70 Low GI: < 40

French bread	136
Instant rice	128
Candy	114
Corn Flakes cereal	110
French fries	107
Honey	104
Carrots	101
Mashed potatoes	100
Whole-wheat bread	97
Soft drinks	97
Chocolate bar	97
Boiled potato	93
White sugar	92
Cheese pizza	86
Pastry	84
White rice	83
Brown rice	78
Bananas	77
Orange juice	74
Oranges	63
Plain yogurt	51
Lentils	42
Cherries	32
Peanut	21

Source: Rick Mendosa. The G.I. Factor, on the Web site http://*www.mendosa.com/sources.htm*

Insulin Kills

How could a hormone (discovered in 1922 by two Canadians, Frederick Banting and John McLeod), which saved millions of insulin-dependent diabetics world-wide now be considered responsible for the so-called civilized diseases?

In fact, in the forties, a certain Dr. Himsworth alerted the medical community on the role of insulin, insulin resistance and hyperinsulinemia as being behind obesity, arteriosclerosis, adult diabetes and heart disease. However, no one followed up on this. It took almost 50 years before this warning resurfaced. Indeed, in 1988, Dr. Reaven made the medical community aware of this phenomenon. Today, it is estimated that every year **half of the deaths** in the Western world are due to excessively high level of insulin in the blood.

Mechanism of Action

Carbohydrates that are eaten are absorbed by the body and end up in the bloodstream. The pancreas immediately reacts and starts secreting insulin, a hormone used to digest sugars by promoting their use by the cells as a source of energy. Therefore, a little sugar causes the secretion of a little insulin; a lot of sugar sharply increases insulin. Gradually, as the blood sugar is digested and its levels are reduced in the blood, insulin lowers as well. When the blood sugar levels become too low, usually four to six hours after a meal, normal hunger is felt and the cycle starts again.

Figure 1. Insulin-carbohydrate mechanism

↑ Carbohydrates	←	↑ Hunger
↓		↑
↑ Insulin → ↓ Blood sugar	→	↓ Insulin

However, under certain conditions, in particular a sedentary lifestyle, obesity, saturated fat intake and heredity, the natural cycle changes. Ingesting carbohydrates thus causes the secretion of insulin, which is no longer effective for digesting sugars (insulin resistance). Sugar-starved cells cry out for it, leading to major sugar cravings. The final result is high levels in the blood of insulin that is not able to digest sugar, a condition known as **hyperinsulinemia**. Paradoxically, at the same time, the blood sugar levels are high, which leads to diabetes and metabolic syndrome complications.

Figure 2. Hyperinsulinemia

↑ Carbohydrates		←			↑	Hunger/snack
↓						↑
↑ Insulin	→ ↑	Blood sugar	→ ↑ ↑	Insulin		

                (cellular resistance)
- Obesity
- Sedentary lifestyle
- Saturated fats
- Genes

Metabolic Syndrome

It was only ten years ago that we recognized this syndrome. The number of symptoms and diseases that are described in this metabolic disorder are caused by too much insulin in the blood. Excessive abdominal body fat, high blood pressure, diabetes, and high levels of cholesterol and triglycerides in the blood are the main signs and they appear in no specific order, generally over a few years. Once this syndrome sets in, its victims develop rampant arteriosclerosis (premature hardening of the arteries).

The main culprit responsible for this secondary hyperinsulinemia is cellular insulin resistance. The only effective treatment is a low-calorie, low-carbohydrate and high-protein diet. With this diet, in less than 48 hours, insulin resistance decreases and the blood sugar levels gradually drop to normal values. But be wary of drugs! They provide a false sense of security and often aggravate the situation in the interim.

Furthermore, in 1993, researchers discovered a gene that promotes this syndrome. If you have a family history of adult diabetes, you probably have this gene. If you keep a healthy weight, exercise regularly and follow the recommendations on pages 22 to 24 in Chapter 1, you will probably never suffer from this syndrome, which is affecting more and more people in our society.

Hypoglycemia

If you have sugar cravings almost every day around the same time, for example, in late afternoon, you probably suffer from hypoglycemia (sugar levels that are too low). Moreover, if you feel a sudden drop in blood sugar, excessive fatigue, have sudden problems concentrating, feel impatient or aggressive, have shaking legs and arms and sweat excessively, and these symptoms seem to diminish with food intake, you probably are suffering from hypoglycemia.

But don't worry. Hypoglycemia is rarely a disease in itself. It is almost always a physiological condition that occurs in people who are genetically susceptible or who have poor dietary habits from eating too much sugar or from having meals more than four hours apart. Once again, insulin is responsible. This is why treating this ailment involves substantially decreasing sugar intake and preferably eating food with high protein content every four hours.

In fact, hyperinsulinemia and hypoglycemia are treated in the same manner.

Sugar Substitutes

What about artificial sweeteners? Now here's a controversial topic. By replacing refined sugar, these substances substantially lower the number of calories absorbed, which is a major benefit. However, we must say that, since they have been on the market, there has been an alarming increase in the number of cases of obesity and diabetes. Is it due to a false sense of security? "If I drink a diet soft drink, I can eat two hamburgers." Or is it due to some unknown physiological mechanism related to the abuse of these substances? We still have no answer to this dilemma.

What I would say in light of our studies on this subject is use sugar substitutes very moderately. The body has very powerful adaptation and survival mechanisms that everyday allow us to survive when exposed to harmful substances or often hostile environmental conditions. What's important is to avoid excessive exposure to them.

By decreasing the use of artificial sweeteners, you will also make it easier to decrease your taste for sugary food.

Chapter 3

Personalized Method

Recent discoveries in nutrition confirm that a moderate, varied and balanced diet is the best measure of good health. There are no miracle foods or foods that you can't eat. If you respect the following guidelines, you will have no difficulty in personalizing your menu to lose weight and maintain a healthy weight.

Your Caloric Requirements

It is easy to evaluate your approximate caloric needs for maintaining the weight that you desire.

For women

It is calculated based on whether you are:

- Sedentary (you do not do any physical activity): Multiply the desired weight by 12 if you are using pounds and by 26 if you are using kilograms;

- Active: Multiply the desired weight by 14 for pounds and by 30 for kilograms;

- Very active (approximately one hour a day of intense physical activity): Multiply the desired weight by 16 for pounds and by 35 for kilograms.

For example: Desired weight: 60 kg, active woman; number of calories per day required to maintain this weight: 60 kg x 30 = 1,800 calories.

For men

It is calculated based on whether you are:

*   Sedentary (you do not do any physical activity): Multiply the desired weight by 14 if you are using pounds and by 30 if you are using kilograms;
*   Active: Multiply the desired weight by 16 for pounds and by 35 for kilograms;
*   Very active (approximately one hour a day of intense physical activity): Multiply the desired weight by 18 for pounds and by 40 for kilograms.

For example: Desired weight: 80 kg, sedentary man; number of calories per day required to maintain this weight: 80 kg x 30 = 2,400 calories.

By doing this calculation, you will have a pretty good idea of your needs. If your weight increases in spite of the fact that you respect these daily numbers, you are probably over-estimating the amount of physical activity you do or under-estimating the amount you eat. If you lose weight, then you have probably underestimated the amount of physical activity or overestimated the number of calories of the food you are eating.

Of course, the above calculations can be adjusted de-pending on the individual. Depending on your needs, you can make any necessary adjustments (higher or lower) by incre-ments of 100 or 200 calories per day.

Your Protein requirements

As we have seen, proteins are the cornerstone for controlling hunger. They must be consumed every four to five hours to en-sure that you feel full (depending on the individual).

To calculate your minimum daily protein requirement, multiply your desired weight in kilograms by 0.8. To convert your weight in pounds into kilograms, divide it by 2.2.

For example: Desired weight: 65 kg; Minimum daily protein requirement to be in good health: 65 kg x 0.8 = 52 g.

If you work out with weights, you can eat even more protein (preferably lean protein), that is up to 1.5 g of protein per kilogram of ideal weight (which is almost double that of a person who does not lift weights).

As well, if you want to lose weight, increase your protein consumption up to 1.5 g of protein for each kilogram of ideal weight for a protein-sparing modified fast. Consult a doctor who specializes in this type of weight-loss plan. Never follow this type of diet without being followed by a competent physician or nurse.

Your Carbohydrate Requirements

Carbohydrates (sugars and other carbohydrates) are required for good health and should provide approximately 50 % of your total calorie intake. However, avoid refined sugars, preferring instead dietary fiber and, if you are susceptible to hypoglycemia and cravings, eat carbohydrates with a source of protein.

Remember that there are carbohydrates (sugars) in most food, especially in milk, vegetables, fruit, bread, cereal, pasta and all starches, legumes and all processed food. Always check labels for this.

To calculate your daily carbohydrate requirements, take the number of calories per day required to maintain your desired weight (by using the formula in "Your Caloric Requirements" on page 33) and divide it by 8.

For example: An active woman weighing 60 kg; Daily carbohydrate requirements: 60 x 30 = 1,800 calories divided by 8 = 225 g of carbohydrates.

To make it easier for you to know the carbohydrate content of different foods, you can evaluate your requirements in units of sugar, using a teaspoon (5 ml) as the reference. Take the number of calories per day that you need to maintain your desired weight (by using the formula in "Your Caloric Requirements" on page 33) and divide it by 32.

For example: An active woman weighing 60 kg; Daily carbohydrate requirements (in teaspoons of sugar): 60 x 30 = 1,800 calories divided by 32 = 56 units (teaspoons of sugar).

Your Fat Requirements

We now know that the human body needs a certain amount of good fat. A person in good health can include 30 % of fat in his or her total daily number of calories. The quality of fat is important: you should consume little saturated fat and a sufficient amount of polyunsaturated and non-hydrogenated fats of vegetable origin. Essential fatty acids, especially omega-3 and omega-6 are preferable.

If you have heart disease, I recommend that you consume only 20 %, or even 10 % of fat; this restriction will help you reduce arteriosclerosis (hardened arteries).

To calculate your daily fat requirements (30 % of calories), take the number of calories that you require to maintain your weight (by using the formula in "Your Caloric Requirements" on page 33) and divide it by 30.

For example, an active man weighing 80 kg; The daily fat requirement: 80 x 35 = 2,800 calories divided by 30 = 840 calories or 93 g of fat.

To make it easier for you to know the fat content of different foods, you can evaluate your need in teaspoons (5 ml) of butter as a reference. Take the number of calories per day that you need to maintain your weight (by using the formula in "Your Caloric Requirements" on page 33) and divide it by 150 to obtain the number of units of fats (teaspoons of butter) that you should not exceed on a daily basis.

For example: An active man weighing 80 kg; Daily fat requirement: 80 x 35 = 2 800 calories divided by 150 = 18.5 units of fat (teaspoons of butter).

Chapter 4

Tips for Motivation and Good Health*

My interest in weight control issues began when I was quite young, as I was the heaviest kid in my class for most of my childhood. My interest and struggles continued through my years of University (including Medical School) and through many years of my medical career as a family doctor. I have my weight under good control now, but it is an "ongoing project".

I limited my medical practice to weight management in 1985. Since that time, I certainly have seen a great number of overweight/obese patients and have acquired a tremendous amount of knowledge and insight into this field... However, the personal miles I have walked have helped me gain a more in depth understanding of the complexity of the disease called "Obesity".

The topics I have chosen to write about in this book are ideas and concepts that I feel have helped countless numbers of patients (including myself) improve their motivation, change their thinking and attitude and ultimately improve their long term weight control success.

SETTING SUCCESS GOALS

I believe most overweight patients set themselves up for failure in that the only goal they have in mind is to reach their "ideal

---

*   Chapter 4 is written by H.J. Lefebre, MD.

weight". At the same time, others around them have put that expectation on them as well (i.e.: their spouse, friends, physicians and society in general). In other words, if someone, for example is 75 lb overweight, everyone feels that person should lose 75 lb to be successful.

Now I'm not saying that an individual can't lose 75 or more pounds, but what if they only lose 30-35 lb? Immediately, they think they have failed, they begin to slip and begin to reinforce that they are indeed a failure and proceed to gain back all their weight and usually more. On the same hand, what if that individual lost their 75 lb, but gained back 5 lb. Again, they feel they have failed at maintenance and begin to gain all their weight back.

I've worked hard with my patients to set "success goals". I advise them to set a goal that for the rest of their life they are going to be below their highest weight. From there it is only a matter of how "successful" they can be. If they lose weight and begin to slip, their positive thoughts will help them turn it around, because they remind themselves of their success. Remember, "success breeds success".

To help convince yourself of this concept, reflect on other areas of your life. In life, if we make some situation better or improve something at home we feel successful and have a sense of accomplishment. It still might not be perfect, but it's better and we're happier. The same should apply to your weight control efforts.

To demonstrate this idea, I've been known to tease a few of my lawyer patients and have asked them to answer yes or no to this question: "Have you been successful in keeping your weight below your highest weight?" They often respond, "Yea, but ...". I then interrupt, "Please just answer the question, yes or no". They smile and say, "Yes, sir".

Once that goal is firmly committed to, set smaller goals (5, 10, 15 lb, etc.). In fact, many medical studies show that a 5-10 % loss of original weight can lead to an improvement in hypertension, diabetes, cholesterol levels, heartburn, energy, etc. The new phrase for improvement in these medical conditions is called "metabolic fitness".

So remember, when setting weight control goals, focus on being below your highest weight for life. You will feel successful, you will talk nice to yourself and will look forward to saying, "Just how good can I get?"

THE DIMMER SWITCH

I first sent this article out in our newsletter several years ago. Since then I have had countless number of patients say that if there was one idea or concept that has helped changed their thinking and attitude in helping with their weight control it has been the **"Dimmer Switch"**. It is for this reason that I thought it would be a good idea to repeat it once again in this book.

It has become apparent to me over the last thirteen years or so, that the majority of overweight patients treat their overweight condition based on whether they are "on" or "off" a diet. Usually they would say to themselves that they have to do something about their weight and would go "on" a diet. They would then proceed to do all the things that are on the "diet on" list (i.e. drink their water, exercise and of course, follow the diet exactly.) This is great, but sooner or later they have a slip. They now say to themselves that I'm "off" the diet and proceed to do all the things that are on the "diet off" list (i.e. eating junk food, stop drinking water, stop exercising etc.). This type of thinking actually sets one up for failure, because the only way to be always "on" is to be always perfect. Since no one can be perfect all the time we'll actually be "off" more than "on". This type of thinking is called "Light Bulb Thinking" because a light bulb is either on or off.

To help combat this problem I get my patients to stop thinking about whether they are on or off a diet and start thinking "weight control". I have them think about weight control as a dimmer switch (that many of us have on the light fixture in our dining rooms.). I get them to analyze a meal, a day, a weekend, a wedding or a party or a stressful event on how much control they had versus whether or not they are on or off their diet. Excellent control would be a very bright light and poor control would be a much fainter light. Keep in mind however that any light is considered control and therefore would demonstrate success. I encourage them to play with their dimmer switch at home at the end of the day and rate their control (even if their family might tease them for doing so).

A wedding

Take a wedding for example. Instead of saying that you are going to go off your diet at the wedding on Saturday night, put the **"Dimmer Switch"** theory into practice. You start off at the wedding by having a couple of cocktails and the light begins to fade (but doesn't go off like the on-off theory.) You catch yourself and eat a few celery sticks instead of potato chips and dip. (The light brightens and you begin to feel positive.) You make various choices from the buffet table causing the light to oscillate back and forth. You dance a lot (exercise) causing a bright light tempered by a few more cocktails (with diet mix) causing the dimmer switch continually to go back and forth. At the end of the evening you summarize the wedding by playing with your dimmer switch at home. All the light on the chandelier would be your success. Just think what would have happened if after your first cocktail the dimmer switch went all the way to off and the light went out. Anytime we shut the light off just think about the power it takes to get the light going again. This is what actually would have happened to our mental powers and motivation when in the past, we practiced the "on-off" diet approach.

In summary, remember the **"Dimmer Switch"** and think **"Weight Control"** versus on or off a diet. Play with your dimmer switch for a few weeks analyzing your day, weekend, happy event (wedding) or a painful, stressful event such as a funeral and remind yourself that as long as there is light shining from the chandelier, you have been successful in controlling your weight.

PREVENTING AND COPING WITH A LAPSE

As I mentioned in my previous newsletter, over the next year I plan on focusing on key concepts that have helped my patients gain better control of their weight problem.

We have talked about setting success goals, the "dimmer switch" and in this article I would like to discuss the concept of preventing and coping with a lapse.

A lapse is simply a term for a deviation from your diet plan, a mistake, a slip, etc. If we continue to slip and string together a series of lapses we relapse back to our previous condition. When a relapse is complete and there is little hope of reversing this negative trend, a collapse has occurred.

To put this concept into practical terms, let's analyze a few common errors in thinking. (For example, let's use a day, a weekend, a week and a holiday).

If we slip at breakfast (e.g. eating a donut) and respond by saying to ourselves, "I've blown the whole day now", and proceed to eat poorly the rest of the day, one small lapse (a 100 calorie donut) can lead to a relapse and ultimately a collapse of the whole day (with perhaps a few thousand extra calories eaten because of our initial response to the first 100 calories).

The same thinking could happen on a weekend. A cocktail and a few snacks on "TGIF" could lead to "there goes the weekend" and who knows how much overeating and drinking could happen then.

Think about Monday morning or the first couple of days on a holiday. If a slip occurred then "there goes the whole week, the holiday, etc".

We can see from the above example that if a lapse occurs and we respond in a negative way, a lapse can automatically lead to collapse. In the following paragraphs let's see how changing our response to our slips can help salvage our day, the weekend, the week and holiday.

An Ounce of Prevention

Throughout our lives we have heard the saying that an ounce of prevention is worth a pound of cure. Therefore, one of the keys to correcting the lapses mentioned in the above paragraphs would be to work on preventing these slips in the first place. However, once the lapse occurs, the most important step would be to learn how to better cope with these lapses and fix the slip right away.

STOP and examine the situation and move to a safe location where you can STAY CALM. If you get anxious and feel guilty, it will only lead to further eating. RENEW YOUR WEIGHT CONTROL GOALS by reminding yourself how far you have progressed and what you still wish to achieve. ANALYSE the SITUATION and learn what triggered the lapse. TAKE CHARGE IMMEDIATELY and don't be afraid to ask for HELP (your partner, co-worker, etc.). I've smiled and told many patients to dial 911 and ask for Dr. Lefebre.

Fix Sooner Than Later

I can't say enough about this concept of coping with a lapse and "fixing it sooner than later" when it comes to someone who has already lost weight (e.g. 50 lb). If they gain back 5 or 10 lb and take action right away they will never gain back 50 lb because they fixed it at 5 or 10. All of us have heard the negative statistics that most people will gain back all of their lost weight, but if we think about it, no one gains back 50-lb overnight. They gain back 1 or 2, then 5, then 10, etc. and if they "fix it sooner than later" they never again will get back to their highest weight. (Obesity has often been described as a disease of procrastination).

So, once again, remember a lapse does not need to lead to a collapse. Try to prevent your slip in the first place, (an ounce of prevention) but if a lapse should occur, TAKE CHARGE IMMEDIATELY and remember the saying we have heard many times in our lives, "FIX IT SOONER THAN LATER". This will allow you to make great strides in having life long success in controlling your weight.

THE SCALE

This might come as a surprise to most of you, but the scale is the number one contributing factor for people quitting their weight control efforts. Yet the factor that leads to most failures is the single most important measurement that everyone focuses on.

I know in our office we weigh patients weekly, but after their weigh-in I bet I spend a third of my time de-emphasizing the scale in an effort to help patients deal with their negative reaction to the scale. I have said countless times to many patients that I would have liked to have run my program without a scale and instead go by improvements in their behavior and feelings, along with improvements in clothing (i.e. passing the "blue-jeans test"). If I would have done this back in 1988 and not had a scale, people would not have understood and most likely my program wouldn't have gotten off the ground. However, thankfully through ongoing counselling and reassurance, a great number of patients have learned to put the scale in its proper perspective.

Think about how often it has happened to you that a week of perfect dieting and vigorous exercise has led to a weight gain on the scale? Your immediate reaction: anger, frustration, despair, and thoughts of quitting. On the other hand what if you deviated a few times that weekend and the scale goes down. The lower scale weight would then reinforce your negative behavior. Therefore your behavior in either case is reinforced by an insensitive machine that didn't ask whether you were wearing different clothes; were having your menstrual cycle;

when your last bowel movement was; whether you were under a lot of stress; whether you drank more or less water than you usually do; performed a lot of exercise or if the weather outside has changed.

All of the above will affect fluid shifts in our body and keep in mind that approximately 70 % of our body is composed of water. I often describe that our body has its own water cycle (similar to the tide in the ocean). The tide comes in and the tide goes out. When we step on the scale we are basically measuring at what stage the tide is at. We can have an hourly tide, a daily tide, a weekly and certainly a monthly tide (as most women will attest to with their menstrual cycles and resultant water retention). All of the above tides can be affected by the factors mentioned in the above paragraph.

The single heaviest factor in our daily, weekly and monthly oral intake is the water we drink. As a test, weigh yourself holding an empty pitcher. Then weigh yourself again with the pitcher containing 12 glasses of water (96oz.). This is the usual recommended daily optimum water intake. The extra weight should be approximately six pounds. What if some of that water is retained over the course of one day? Naturally, the scale will go up. Then try filling a big bucket with an entire weeks supply of water. This should weigh over 40 lb This is the weight of water alone that you would drink in a week and should some of that water be retained, again, the scale will go up (even if you have lost body fat and your clothes feel looser.) Some of you might think from the above examples that if you were to retain some of the water it would be best not to drink as much. The opposite is true. Remember, the *more* water you drink the *less* you retain.

Another area where the scale affects most patients is when they know that they have gained weight (e.g. after a holiday, or after a month has gone by between visits to the office). They fear coming in to the office to weigh and often continue to procrastinate returning day after day, week after week. They feel guilty, ashamed, and worry about what we might think about their weight gain. Again over the years I have told countless numbers of patients that they do not have to worry about weighing-in. Just get back to the office for a friendly, encouraging visit and some positive reassurance. They can get on the scale whenever they are ready. Likewise, if after repeated visits, a patient is still very uptight about the scale, we get them to avoid weighing for a while and get them to focus on their positive behavior and attitude. I can't emphasize enough that the focus of our program is not the scale... the focus is on you, your behavior, attitudes and feelings.

The key to weight control is changing your behavior. Improving your behavior will lead to good feelings about yourself, causing better compliance with your eating and exercise plan, which will translate into noticeable inches lost in your clothing. As a last measure of success, check the scale. It will take practice, but one of the biggest favors you can do for yourself to achieve long lasting weight control success is to learn to put the scale in its place... and many times perhaps, the best place for the scale is out the window.

CALORIE BANKING

Once patients have reached maintenance, "calorie banking" is a concept that is a very practical approach in helping them balance their food intake for life. It stems from the idea that we live in a society that is basically 5 days on and 2 days off (referring to a work or school week).

Once a patient has lost weight and wishes to go on maintenance, their caloric food intake is slowly increased to 1200 calories for women and 1500 for men. At this time we start to talk about the calorie banking principle.

Let's say that a female patient has lost down to 130 lb. Her approximate caloric needs to maintain this weight would be 1700-1800 cal. If we were to increase her intake to that level, there would be no room for extras (as we all know, it is usually the extras that are responsible for weight gain). Once we outline the 1200 cal. plan we get our patients, over the following week, to see if there would be any extra food choices they would like to add to this (for example, another bread serving which would add about 70 calories). We need this input because we want them to feel that their food intake will be adequate for the five regular days of the week. This would work out to be about 400-500 cal. per day less that they would need to maintain their weight. We now transfer this 2000-2500 cal. (representing five days) into a theoretical calorie bank that they can spend and draw from on the weekend (or any other times during the week when they have extras).

Basically therefore it is a way to balance your "food intake account" for the week, just like you would balance a real bank account.

For men, we apply the same principle but use a 1500 cal. diet as a base.

Please note:

Always keep in mind that these numbers are approximate, but it's understanding and applying the basic "calorie banking" principle that is important. We also strongly emphasize to our patients the importance of ongoing maintenance visits (weekly at first, then every 2 weeks, then three weeks and finally monthly) to ensure that the "calorie banking" idea is working for them.

Weight maintenance is a life-long balancing act. In all reality, we have to work on balancing our food intake (i.e. Energy Intake), our activity and exercise (i.e. Energy Expenditure) and our water intake for life. Above all, we have to keep our attitude and motivation positive (I always say that the best exercise of all, is to keep our head going!). I'm confident that applying the above ideas including the "Calorie Banking" principle will be key factors in your life long weight control success.

REALISTIC GOALS

This topic is somewhat of an overlap to previous newsletters (setting success goals, dimmer switch and coping with a lapse), but setting day to day realistic goals warrants its own discussion.

Humans in general and dieters in particular, tend to be perfectionists and as a result try to be perfect all the time. If they slip on their diet they feel guilty and suffer from a loss of self worth which often sets off a negative vicious cycle of overeating.

The negative emotional response usually occurs as a result of initial goal setting. If we say that we will never slip on a diet and a slip occurs, we feel guilty which often leads to thoughts about giving up and quitting. If we expect to exercise every day and we miss one day, once again, failure thoughts occur, leading to wanting to give up exercise altogether. In addition, expectations to lose weight each week sets one up for discouragement, self-blame and thoughts of "throwing in the towel" if the scale doesn't go down every week.

Working more with realism than perfectionism has helped a great many of my patients. Learning to set more realistic goals in the first place is a key for preventing negative guilt feelings. (Remember: Guilt is often measured by the difference between the goal that we set and the degree of achievement of that goal).

Changing, "I will never slip" to, "I will follow the diet the best I can", leads to satisfaction and a desire to do even better. Instead of a rigid goal of exercising every day, try increasing your level of activity at your own level and pace. You will find that the increase is steady and you will feel a sense of pride in doing something positive. Instead of expecting weight loss every week, accept a more realistic goal of perhaps a loss ten out of twelve weeks. You will realize that you will lose weight most weeks and will feel good about your hard work.

Once again, by being realistic, you have a great chance of achieving your goals. You will break the negative guilty vicious cycle, feel good about yourself and make a significant positive impact in your weight control efforts.

SUCCESSFUL RESTARTING STARTS
WITH DECREASING GUILT

After an absence from attending our office, many of you hold back returning because of guilt or embarrassment that you have regained some weight. We are quite aware of this and as a result continue to pass on many reassuring ideas that have helped our restart patients deal with much of their guilt and negative self talk. This in turn has helped steer them back on the right course. Many times I have said that I should have a blinking neon sign at our front office door that says: **"Leave your guilt outside and come on in."**

Following are key concepts that will help reassure you, decrease your guilt and get you back on the right track:

REMEMBER:

1. It takes a lot of courage to restart. It is human nature to feel guilty, to think that we have let ourselves or others down. Therefore, taking this first step is a tremendous accomplishment.

2. Working at controlling your weight can be the toughest challenge in your life. Try to refer to it as your life long project versus a battle, struggle, etc. You will get more positive results because *you* are a very important project and worth working on.

3. A weight condition is a "chronic one" similar to high blood pressure, diabetes, multiple sclerosis, rheumatoid arthritis, etc. In these conditions, there are times when there is good control and times when there are flare-ups (i.e. the condition worsens).

4. Strive for control not cure. Keep applying my dimmer switch principle.

5. Understanding the complexity of a weight problem greatly lessens your guilt. I have a saying: one symptom brings our patients in-they are overweight but in reality

there maybe 1001 reasons that contribute to this one symptom.

6. Never Quit. If you never quit on your weight control efforts again, you will never have to restart.

7. Fix sooner than later. If you have lost weight and restart still below your highest weight, you have been successful.

8. Learn from your mistakes and slips and improve on the reasons that led to your weight regain.

9. If you are on a plateau, convert the "dreaded plateau" into a learning opportunity. Many times the best maintainers are those who lose in a stepwise fashion: they lose some weight then maintain, lose more, then maintain, etc.

10. Identify any mental or motivational blocks standing in your way. Read Dr. Larocque's book: Be Thin Through Motivation.

11. Review and retake the Mental Weight test. Many people will regain their weight if their mental weight is high. The ideal is to have your desired physical weight and your mental weight be the same.

12. I'll often say that there is good news and bad news to your weight condition. The bad news is that you will always have a weight problem. The good news is that if you accept it and deal with it in a proper fashion, you won't be overweight again.

I will continue to pass on more tidbits that (since 1988) have helped our patients understand the complexity of their weight problem and have helped lessen their guilt and negative feelings about themselves. This in turn has had a very favorable impact on their weight control success.

"TREAT" VS "CHEAT"

How often have you said to yourself that you "cheated" on your diet because you had a piece of cheesecake? No doubt this resulted in guilty feelings, self-punishment and contributed to lower self-image thoughts about yourself. In fact I'm sure many times the self-punishment ended up leading to more over-eating and a vicious bingeing cycle. These negative thoughts and actions stem from the guilt that arose from the fact that you felt that you "cheated" on your diet. It is a fact in life that when you cheat someone or do wrong, and you are caught, a form of punishment is handed out. This is what you do to yourself when you feel you "cheated" by having a piece of cheesecake.

I have told countless number of patients over the years that when they would like to have a little dessert, for example, change the word "cheat" to "treat". This will break the guilt vicious cycle, because you are telling yourself that you are "treating" yourself and as a result, good feelings and thoughts will come about.

Some patients have been worried that they might convince themselves that they can have dessert anytime because they will want to treat themselves all the time. I believe this won't happen because you will know that doing it all the time is not a treat – this behavior would revert back to being a bad habit. Remember a "treat" is a special event, occasion or a pleasure given.

Another way of remembering this concept is in this catchy phrase: If you "legalize" you will "equalize". In other words, if something is allowed, and it is all right to do it, no guilty feelings will result. You will feel good about your little "treat" and carry on with positive thoughts about your weight control efforts.

So, from now on, throw away those guilt thoughts by remembering to convert "cheat" to "treat" when you have that "little extra". One last comment: both "tr*eat*" and "ch*eat*" have the word *EAT* in it. *(Very interesting!!!)*

TRIPLE "A" PROCESS FOR POSITIVE CHANGE

How many times have all of us asked ourselves why we get this uncontrollable urge to eat when we get upset over something (and of course many times we give in to this urge). Numerous patients over the years have asked me the same question. There isn't a simple answer but when I am posed this question I usually pull out a little slip of paper and write down three words under each other beginning with the letter "A":

Awareness
Acceptance
Action

To make changes in our life we have to go through this "AAA" process. We first have to become "**Aware**" of why we do the things we do. (As the saying goes you're half way there when you become aware of the problem). We actually begin to associate food with our emotions long before we are even aware of it. It all starts as a baby when we cried and got fed. Then when we were a one-year-old and had our first bleeding nose (and after we were all cleaned up) we got a cookie or an ice cream cone to "make us feel better". This nurturing our emotions with food continued through our lives as we got older and our problems got bigger. Becoming aware of this association with food and our emotions is the first step to change, because it truly makes sense when you reflect back in your life and analyze it in a proper manner.

The next step for change is "**Acceptance**". We have to go through this step before we can perform the right "Action".We have to accept that this is what happened when we were young and how we were raised. We have to also accept that we are all human and that we have these human qualities. Willingness to accept these things allows our guilt feelings to decrease and consequently our stress level goes down. This in turn will enable us to think things through in a calmer, methodical manner resulting in better decisions being made. If we don't go through the acceptance phase properly and we keep denying our past, keep blaming others for how we act, or we keep refusing to accept that we are all human, we won't be able to take the next step in a correct fashion. However, if we go through the first two stages properly we're ready to proceed to the next phase "Action".

The right course of "**Action**" is to begin using positive self-talk (affirmations) and avoid the negatives. Negative self-talk such as "why can't I just get control of myself" or "what's the matter with me" only increases your guilt and reinforces your negative behavior. Use positive affirmations such as "I accept myself and other people and things for who or what they are" or "I'm in control of my emotions and I eat well, I'm proud of myself and I to like reward myself positively". This positive self-talk should be followed by your mental movie visualizing yourself performing your new positive course of action.

Looking at weight control in general, one certainly has to apply the "AAA" process to be successful. Many people often jump right to the "Action" phase and think that the first thing to do when they need to lose weight is to go on a diet. When the diet is over and they gain their weight back they blame the diet or feel like a failure and the vicious yo-yo cycle starts. An overweight person has to go through all 3 phases. They have to become aware of the complexity of their problem and that it will require a life long commitment to be successful. They have to accept these challenges and then they are ready to take the proper action: a proper diet, increased activity (physical exercise) and water drinking, all combined with a positive attitude and self-talk (motivational exercise).

Applying the "Triple A" process of "**Awareness, Acceptance & Action**" in the future not only will improve your weight control success but will assist you in making positive changes whenever the need arises throughout the rest of your life.

TAKING CARE OF "NUMERO UNO"

Over the last 12 years or so, I've lost count on how many times that I've heard a patient say, "I just don't have time for myself". At the same time when these same patients do come in, they often feel guilty that they are taking time for themselves or are spending time and money that could go towards other obligations (e.g. kids, spouses etc...). As well, I have caught many

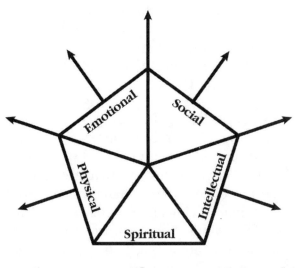

Dimensions of Optimal Health

patients nodding off to sleep while they wait for me because often their visit to see us is the only time they have to themselves. When this type of dialogue or situation takes place during an office visit, I pull out the following little diagram from my desk drawer and start to talk about taking care of "Numero Uno".

The diagram pictured above represents you ("Numero Uno") and your five dimensions of optimal health. The physical triangle, of course, represents our body and the other four triangles represent what takes place above the shoulders in our mind (these four triangles contributing to make us all the complex creatures that we are). In fact, during our life, whether we are aware of it or not, we are striving to keep all of the five triangles in balance.

Most people think they come in to see me to fix the physical triangle because they only have one symptom and that is, they have a weight problem. However, once I show them this diagram, they soon realize there are perhaps 1001 reasons behind this one physical symptom (the 1001 reasons stemming from the other four triangles). Interesting to note here, is that when one says, "that does it, I'm going to do something about my weight", weight loss, and weight control actually start in the mind, therefore, taking care of the physical triangle takes place in the mind as well.

The arrows surrounding the triangles represent all the factors that we deal with in our lives: Our spouse, children, other family members and other commitments (volunteering, committee obligations etc.). For many, there are several more arrows that can be added to this diagram. If one thinks about these arrows as energy being pulled or taken away from each of the triangles, the triangles (or "Numero Uno") could shrink until they are nothing but a speck on the paper that you can hardly see. This is why I emphasize that each and everyone of us has to take care of "Numero Uno" first. Right away I can hear you say (as I have heard many say) that this is being selfish and these type of feelings could lead to a lot of guilt. I reply by mentioning that truly selfish people are egocentric, step on others to get their way or put others down to rise to the top and these type of people do not feel guilt. An individual who truly takes care of themselves in a positive way and is balancing out the five triangles is kind, considerate, charitable, energetic and has a lot of energy to give to others. (Without suffering from guilt!).

My simple advice to you is to take care of yourself first ("Numero Uno") and keep the triangles at full size. Picture all of the arrows revolving around you and your full size triangles. Think of the arrows as energy to give, rather than someone or something taking energy from you. As well, imagine the arrows extending out from you in a positive manner (like open arms) with yourself giving out this newfound energy. Compare this to a negative picture of having the arrows represent someone or something pulling away at you and exhausting your energy stores (and as stated above, the triangles becoming nothing but a speck on the piece of paper). Continuing to take time for yourself and working on this "Numero Uno" principle will help you feel good about "you" in general and as well, go a long way in contributing to your weight control success.

DIET SABOTEURS

How often have the following examples happened to you?: 1) You've lost a lot of weight and suddenly a co-worker brings in donuts to the office. 2) Your husband brings home a box of your favorite chocolates to celebrate your weight loss. 3) Your Mom bakes your favorite pie and tells you how great you look. 4) Your friend tells you not to lose any more weight because your face is looking quite gaunt. 5) A cousin who hasn't seen you for months makes a big fuss over your weight loss in front of a big crowd at a party. After that you notice a drop in your motivation.

Believe it or not the above examples are constantly taking place. Since I began my bariatric practice in Calgary back in 1988, I have found the area of diet sabotaging to be one of the most intriguing challenges a "dieter" has to face and a subject that caught me a little by surprise when I first began in the weight control field.

"Diet Saboteurs" fall into 4 main categories: IGNO-RANCE, MEANNESS, GUILT and JEALOUSY. The examples in the first paragraph could be any or all of the four categories. Ignorance is a harsh word but it simply means a lack of knowledge, awareness or understanding. You wouldn't want to call your Mom "ignorant" when she bakes you a pie but she simply wants to show you how much she loves you and isn't aware a pie is not the treat you desire. People might say that you look gaunt because they have a picture of you with a round face. When that picture changes (your face gets thinner) they subconsciously might perceive it as a negative when in fact your thinner face makes you look better and healthier (certainly not gaunt). Interestingly enough, these same people would notice someone's face get rounder when they were gaining weight and probably comment on that as well.

Bringing in donuts could be a mean attempt to get you off your diet. It could also be an act of jealousy or a result of guilt feelings (because they have been unable to control their weight, if you eat a donut this would make them feel better). A husband giving chocolates could be showing you his love but he might lack the understanding that food treats are what you don't desire at this time. The chocolates also could represent that he might feel threatened or jealous over your new looks, success and newfound attention.

On the opposite side of the fence, getting compliments could lead to a drop in motivation for various reasons, one simply being that we think we're okay now and don't need to lose any more weight. Getting compliments in public could lead to one's uneasiness and thus people giving compliments could unknowingly be diet saboteurs.

To combat diet saboteurs, first of all memorize the four categories (if you haven't already). Learn to know why people around you are doing what they are doing and in what category they fall into (realizing that being mean, acting jealous or feeling guilty are their problems and don't allow them to get the best of you). Write down polite but firm responses that you might use next time a situation arises. Rehearse and practice them, so that the next time, you will be ready. Reassure Mom that you know she loves you, but you feel great, your diet is going well and she can help you by letting you eat what is best for you. When one of the partners in a relationship loses weight it can change the dynamics of the partnership. A lot of understanding and reassurance may need to be given by both partners and a reminder to your spouse that flowers instead of chocolates would make a great gift.

It's hard enough dealing with your own pressures to stay with your diet let alone pressures from others. Nevertheless, it is a fact that diet saboteurs do exist. However, by becoming more aware of people's actions around us and working on ways to combat difficult situations, will help you make great strides in your weight control success.

"TOUGHEST CHALLENGE OF ONE'S LIFE"

I don't know how many times I have heard patients say, "I wonder why I can't get my weight under control" or "I can't figure out why I can't lose weight". They then go on to say that they quit smoking, they gave up drinking and that they are successful in most other areas in their life (their marriage, family life, their careers, etc.). They are just unable to come up with the answer.

My first response is to mention that a smoker has to use the all or nothing control method. They stop smoking (you are either a smoker or a non-smoker). An alcoholic must stop drinking. However, you just can't stop eating. We have to use other methods to control our weight and this is generally harder than the all or nothing method described above.

Secondly, I will often remind them that losing weight might appear to be one thing, but in reality we all know that a weight problem is a very complex issue and perhaps is the end result of 1001 reasons or events that have occurred in an individuals life (previously described in my "Taking care of Numero Uno" newsletter).

I will often liken your weight control journey as climbing a mountain. What if your friend asked you if you would like to climb Mount Rundle (a famous mountain in Banff) next Saturday. You thought that sounded like fun. When Saturday came, you put on your best walking boots, grabbed a warm coat, a pair of gloves and away you went. You started up the mountain and you soon realized that this was way harder than you thought. You gave up and came back down. You now have two options: Forget the whole mountain climbing idea or you become even more determined to get to the top. You begin visualizing yourself at the summit. You start a vigorous training program, and acquire the correct mountain gear, etc. In other words, you became aware of the tremendous challenge ahead and you worked on your motivation and determination and acquired the right tools to become successful.

Taking on a weight loss, weight control challenge is very similar. For most, it is the *"Toughest challenge of one's life"*. We all have to become aware of this, accept the effort it is going to take and then take the appropriate action. (Again refer back to my "AAA" newsletter on awareness, acceptance and action). Keep in mind that there is one important difference between climbing a mountain and a weight control problem. Dealing with your weight problem is not a one-time event of just getting there – **a weight control challenge lasts a lifetime**. We all have to continue to work on our attitude, motivation, eating habits, water drinking and physical activity for the rest of our life.

When patients are struggling with their motivation, I'll often give them a sheet to fill out to help them get "to the top". I get them to fill in at least 12 reasons why they want to lose weight and maintain their weight loss. To help them further, I get them to think that they will wake up the next morning and will have "won their goal weight" and all the benefits that go with it (similar to a list they would make if they were asked to write down what they would do with the money from winning the "6/49 lotto".). I get them to visualize realistic goals, experience them in their mind and savor the feelings as if they were real. I then get them to transfer these very positive goals and feelings on to what I call my "Tug of War" sheet. The left side of the sheet asks all the reasons why they want to get control of their weight and the right side asks why you can't or don't want to get control. Putting it down on paper in this manner will give a clear picture of your internal struggles and what forces are winning the "Tug of war". This will also help identify a person's mental blocks. I also refer them to Dr. Larocque's book, "Be Thin through Motivation" to help them identify and deal with these mental blocks.

Once again then, motivation is the key to your success. Working on the ideas, such as those I have mentioned above, will help you become successful in your life long weight control journey and go a long way in helping you finally get "over the top".

PART TWO

Recipes that will satisfy your hunger

In the following pages, you will find over 250 healthful recipes so that you can control your weight without feeling hungry.

They will help you reduce your risk for cancer, hardening of the arteries (poor circulation), heart disease, diabetes and hypertension, as well as decrease your blood cholesterol and triglyceride levels.

All in all, these succulent recipes will help keep you healthy.

Make the ones you like the most on a regular basis. Soon they will become part of your life.

Bon appétit and stay healthy without feeling hungry.

Lamb with Orange

Combine orange juice with ginger, salt and pepper. Add lamb. Let marinate for 2 hours. Remove meat from marinade. Meanwhile cook the onion in a non-stick pan. Add meat and brown rapidly. Pour marinade into a baking dish. Then add chicken broth and heat until it boils. Add the meat and the onion. Bake at 325 °F/160 °C for 30 minutes. Add broth if necessary. Garnish with orange slice and parsley. Makes 1 serving.

Lamb, cubed	4 oz (120 ml)
Orange juice, unsweetened	1 tbsp (15 ml)
Onion, minced	2 tbsp (30 ml)
Chicken broth	¼ cup (60 ml)
Ginger	¼ tsp (1 ml)
Orange, sliced	1 slice
Parsley	
Salt and pepper	1 pinch

For 1 serving:
Carbohydrates: 5 g = 1 unit
Fat: 11 g = 2 units
Proteins: 24 g
Calories: 220

❖

Lamb Brochettes

In a deep pan, mix the tomato juice, the yogurt, the mustard, the powdered mint, the shallots, salt, pepper and cinnamon. Marinate the meat in the sauce for 4 hours. On metal skewers place the meat, mushrooms, tomatoes, peppers and onions. Broil in oven or on barbecue. Occasionally turn the brochettes and brush them with remaining sauce. Makes 2 servings.

Tomato juice	2 tbsp (30 ml)
Plain yogurt, 2 %	¼ cup (60 ml)
Mustard, dry	1 tsp (5 ml)
Shallot, chopped	1 tsp (5 ml)
Cinnamon	1 pinch
Lamb cubes (1 ½")(3.5 cm)	8 oz (240 g)
Fresh mushrooms	8
Tomato quarters	1
Green pepper	½ cup (125 ml)
Onion	1
Mint, powdered	1 tsp (5 ml)
Curcuma	½ tsp (2 ml)
Curry, powder	1 tsp (1 ml)
Salt	¼ tsp (1 ml)
Black pepper	1 pinch

For one serving:

Carbohydrates:	12 g = 3 units
Fat:	7 g = 1.5 units
Proteins:	26 g
Calories:	228

❖

Lamb Loaf

Mix all ingredients and pour into a small oven dish. Bake at 350 °F (180 °C) for 15 minutes or more. Makes 2 servings.

Ground lamb, cooked	6 oz (180 g)
Oatmeal	1 tbsp (15 ml)
Egg, beaten	1
Chicken broth	¼ cup (60 ml)
Fresh parsley, chopped	1 tsp (5 ml)
Marjoram	¼ tsp (1 ml)
Clove garlic, chopped	1
Salt and black pepper, to taste	

For one serving:
Carbohydrates: 4 g = 1 unit
Fat: 11 g = 2 units
Proteins: 28 g
Calories: 232

❖

Italian Steak

Cut meat into thin strips and put in baking dish. Add all other ingredients except salt. Microwave, covered, at full power for 4 minutes. Add a little salt and pepper. Serve. Makes 1 serving.

Beef minute steak	4 oz (120 g)
Tomato sauce	2 tbsp (30 ml)
Mozzarella skimmed cheese, grated milk	1 tbsp (15 ml)
Mustard dried	¼ tsp (1 ml)
Italian seasoning	½ tsp (2 ml)
White wine	½ tsp (2 ml)
Fresh mushrooms, minced	2
Salt and black pepper, to taste	

For one serving:
Carbohydrates: 7 g = 2 units
Fat: 10 g = 2 units
Proteins: 31 g
Calories: 241

❖

Oriental Steak

Brown the meat in a non-stick pan. Drain well and add onion, garlic, green pepper, celery and broth. Season and cover. Let simmer on low heat for 20 minutes (do not boil). Add soy sauce and simmer 5 more minutes. Serve. Makes 2 servings.

Beef, cut into thin strips	8 oz (240 g)
Onion, thinly chopped	2 tbsp (30 ml)
Garlic clove, crushed	1
Green pepper, cut into thin strips	1 cup (250 ml)
Fresh celery, cut	½ cup (125 ml)
Consommé (beef)	½ cup (125 ml)
Soy sauce, sugar free	1 tsp (5 ml)
Salt and black pepper, to taste	

For one serving:

Carbohydrates:	11 g = 3 units
Fat:	6 g = 1 unit
Proteins:	27 g
Calories:	213

❖

Pepper Steak

Brush the steak on both sides with sauce. Sprinkle peppercorns all over the steak. Use fingers to get more peppercorns on steak. Microwave at full power for 30 seconds. Steak should be medium-cooked. Makes 1 serving.

Beef steak, lean cut	4 oz (120 g)
Worcestershire sauce	1 tsp (5 ml)
Peppercorns, to taste	

For one serving:
Carbohydrates: 0 g
Fat: 6 g = 1 unit
Proteins: 26 g
Calories: 169

❖

Green Pepper Steak

Season steak with salt, onion powder and black pepper. Brown in skillet, then add water and let simmer until tender. Add consommé, onions and more water. Simmer covered for about 10 minutes. Makes 1 serving.

Beef, round steak	4 oz (120 g)
Onion, chopped	1 cup (250 ml)
Consommé (onion)	1 tsp (5 ml)
Green pepper, sliced	1
Water	2 tbsp (30 ml)

For one serving:
Carbohydrates: 29 g = 7 units
Fat: 8 g = 1.5 units
Proteins: 31 g
Calories: 310

Isabelle Steak

Cut all visible fat from beef and discard. Place steak in a microwave container used to cook meat. Microwave at full power for 1 minute.

SAUCE:

In a small bowl, mix plain yogurt, mustard, wine vinegar, shallot and Worcestershire sauce. Salt and pepper to taste. Microwave at full power for 10 to 15 seconds. Serve with steak. Makes 1 serving.

Beef fillet	4 oz (120 g)
Plain yogurt	2 tbsp (30 ml)
Dijon mustard	1 tsp (5 ml)
Wine vinegar	½ tsp (2 ml)
Shallot, chopped	1
Worcestershire sauce	few drops
Salt, to taste	
Black pepper, to taste	

For one serving:
Carbohydrates: 3 g = 0.5 unit
Fat: 7 g = 1.5 units
Proteins: 27 g
Calories: 189

Swiss Steak

Place steak in baking dish. Add all other ingredients. Microwave at medium-high (70 %) for 20 minutes. Let stand 5 minutes. Add a little salt and pepper. Sprinkle with parsley and serve. Makes 1 serving.

Beef sirloin	4 oz (120 g)
Green pepper, minced	¼ cup (60 ml)
Onion, minced	¼ cup (60 ml)
Tomatoes (canned)	2
Tomato paste	1 tsp (5 ml)
Fresh mushrooms, minced	3
Parsley, chopped	1 tbsp (15 ml)
Salt and black pepper, to taste	

For one serving:
Carbohydrates: 19 g = 5 units
Fat: 7 g = 1.5 units
Proteins: 28 g
Calories: 242

❖

Country Casserole

In a non-stick pan, cook shallots and garlic. Remove them and then brown the meat. Set aside. In casserole, cook tomatoes, add salt, pepper and broth. Bring to a boil and add meat, garlic and shallots. Cover and let simmer on low heat for 1 hour. Add mushrooms and cook for 15 minutes. Before serving, garnish with parsley. Makes 2 servings.

Beef, cubed lean cut	8 oz (240 g)
Shallot, chopped	2 tbsp (30 ml)
Tomatoes, peeled	½ cup (125 ml)
Garlic clove, chopped	1
Consommé (beef), fat free	½ cup (125 ml)
Fresh mushrooms, sliced	½ cup (125 ml)
Parsley and black pepper, to taste	
Salt	½ tsp (2 ml)

For one serving:

Carbohydrates:	4 g = 1 unit
Fat:	9 g = 2 units
Proteins:	26 g
Calories:	200

❖

Cantonese Beef

Place meat, green pepper, onion and garlic in baking dish. Cover and microwave at full power for 1 ½ minutes. Add all others ingredients except tomato. Cover and microwave at 70 % (medium-high) for 3 minutes. Add tomato. Cover and let stand 5 minutes. Add salt and pepper before serving. Makes 1 serving.

Beef, in strips lean cut	4 oz (120 g)
Green pepper, minced	½
Tomatoes wedges	2
Ginger, fresh	1 slice
Onion, chopped	1 tbsp (15 ml)
Garlic clove, chopped	1
Consommé, fat free (beef)	2 tbsp (30 ml)
Soy sauce, sugar free	1 tsp (5 ml)
Salt and black pepper, to taste	

For one serving:

Carbohydrates:	18 g = 4.5 units
Fat:	14 g = 3 units
Proteins:	34 g
Calories:	329

❖

Cream and Mushrooms Beef

Broil beef fillet briefly (until it is still rare). In a non-stick pan, brown onion and garlic for 2 minutes. Add mushrooms and cook for 3 minutes, stirring occasionally. Sprinkle vegetables with flour and mix rapidly. Stir in broth. Add tomato paste and let cook until it thickens, stirring often. Remove pan from heat. Add yogurt, pepper and parsley, mix well. Add meat and cook until hot. Serve over hot, cooked rice. Makes 2 servings.

Beef fillet	8 oz (240 g)
Onion, chopped	2 tbsp (30 ml)
Garlic clove, chopped	1
Fresh mushrooms, sliced	1 cup (250 ml)
Flour	1 tbsp (15 ml)
Consommé, fat free (beef)	¾ cup (180 ml)
Tomato paste	2 tsp (10 ml)
Plain yogurt, 2 %	½ cup (125 ml)
Parsley, chopped	1 tbsp (15 ml)
Rice, cooked	1 cup (250 ml)
Black pepper	1 pinch

For one serving:

Carbohydrates:	47 g	= 12 units
Fat:	15 g	= 3 units
Proteins:	39 g	
Calories:	482	

❖

Beef and Carrots

Place carrots, onion, water and consommé in microwave dish. Microwave, covered, at full power for 5 minutes. Add meat, tomato sauce and thyme. Microwave, covered, at medium-high for 5 minutes. Add salt, pepper and let stand 5 minutes before serving. Makes 1 serving.

Beef minute steak   4 oz (120 g)
Carrot, sliced   ½ cup (125 ml)
Onion, chopped   1 tbsp (15 ml)
Water   ¼ cup (60 ml)
Tomato sauce   2 tbsp (30 ml)
Consommé, fat free (beef)   ½ tsp (2 ml)
Thyme   ¼ tsp (1 ml)
Salt and black pepper, to taste

For one serving:
Carbohydrates: 18 g = 4.5 units
Fat: 14 g = 3 units
Proteins: 32 g
Calories: 328

❖

Vegetables and Beef

Sauté cauliflower and onion in non-stick pan for 5 minutes. Add beef, beans, spices and consommé. Cook and stir 5 more minutes or until meat is brown and beans are tender-crisp. Makes 1 serving.

Beef in thin strips lean cut	4 oz (120 g)
Cauliflower, thinly chopped	½ cup (125 ml)
Onion, chopped	2 tbsp (30 ml)
Green beans, cut (or frozen)	½ cup (125 ml)
Savory	½ tsp (2 ml)
Sage	½ tsp (2 ml)
Consommé onion (fat free)	2 tbsp (30 ml)

For one serving:

Carbohydrates:	8 g = 2 units
Fat:	13 g = 2.5 units
Proteins:	32 g
Calories:	281

❖

Beef with Vegetables, traditional oven

Broil beef cubes until they are slightly browned. Put in baking dish and add all other ingredients. Bake at 325 °F/160 °C for 30 to 45 minutes. Makes 2 servings.

Beef cubed lean cut	8 oz (240 g)
Consommé (beef)	¼ cup (60 ml)
Bean sprouts	1 cup (250 ml)
Carrot, sliced	½ cup (125 ml)
Cabbage, sliced	½ cup (125 ml)
Onion, chopped	¼ cup (60 ml)
Fresh celery, shredded	½ cup (125 ml)
Green pepper	¼ cup (60 ml)
Thyme	½ tsp (2 ml)
Basil	½ tsp (2 ml)
Garlic clove, minced	1
Salt and black pepper, to taste	

For one serving:

Carbohydrates:	24 g = 6 units	
Fat:	14 g = 3 units	
Proteins:	35 g	
Calories:	351	

❖

Beef and Vegetables, microwave

Microwave beef at medium-high (70 %) for 4 minutes. Add water and consommé and microwave at the same power for 6 minutes. Add vegetables and microwave again at the same power for 8 minutes more. Let stand 5 minutes before serving. Makes 1 serving.

Beef, lean and cubed	4 oz (120 g)
Green pepper	¼ cup (60 ml)
Fresh celery	¼ cup (60 ml)
Cauliflower	½ cup (125 ml)
Broccoli	½ cup (125 ml)
Onion, chopped	1 tbsp (15 ml)
Water	1 cup (250 ml)
Consommé, fat free (beef)	1 tsp (5 ml)
Salt and black pepper, to taste	

For one serving:

Carbohydrates:	16 g	= 4 units
Fat:	14 g	= 3 units
Proteins:	38 g	
Calories:	333	

❖

Chinese Beef with Tomatoes

In a bowl, combine soy sauce and wine vinegar. Mix beef strips with mixture and let marinate for 1 hour. In a non-stick pan, cook marinated beef with the onions, garlic and green pepper slices for 2-3 minutes. Add marinade, water, beef consommé and tomato wedges. Cook for 5 to 7 minutes and serve very hot. Makes 1 serving.

Beef, in thin strips lean cut	4 oz (120 g)
Wine vinegar	2 tbsp (30 ml)
Soy sauce, sugar free	2 tbsp (30 ml)
Onion, cut	1
Garlic clove, crushed	1
Green pepper, in strips	½ cup (125 ml)
Tomato, fresh	1
Water	¼ cup (60 ml)
Consommé (beef)	½ tsp (2 ml)

For one serving:
Carbohydrates: 23 g = 6 units
Fat: 7 g = 1.5 units
Proteins: 27 g
Calories: 259

❖

Braised Beef with Carrots

Cut the beef into thin strips. In a non-stick pan, slightly cook the beef. Add carrot slices, tomato paste, beef consommé, water, salt, pepper, and fine herbs. Cover and cook on medium heat for 1 hour. Place meat in serving dish surrounded with carrot slices. Makes 1 serving.

Beef, lean cut	4 oz (120 g)
Carrot, sliced	1 cup (250 ml)
Tomato paste	1 tsp (5 ml)
Consommé, fat free (beef)	1 tsp (5 ml)
Water	¾ cup (180 ml)

Thyme, parsley, salt and black pepper, to taste

For one serving:	
Carbohydrates:	25 g = 6 units
Fat:	8 g = 1.5 units
Proteins:	27 g
Calories:	274

❖

Fine Herbs Patty

First mix fine herbs, then shape the beef into a patty. Coat patty with the herbs and cook in a non-stick pan for 3 to 5 minutes on both sides. Add a little salt and pepper. Makes 1 serving.

Beef, lean ground	4 oz (120 g)
Tarragon, to taste	
Parsley, to taste	
Salt, to taste	
Black pepper, to taste	

For one serving:	
Carbohydrates:	0 g
Fat:	17 g = 3.5 units
Proteins:	21 g
Calories:	242

Surprise Ground Steak

Combine all ingredients in a mixing bowl and shape into a patty. Microwave at full power for 1 minute, turning patty over during cooking. Let stand 1 minute before serving. Makes 1 serving.

Beef, lean ground	4 oz (120 g)
Fresh mushrooms, chopped	1 tbsp (15 ml)
Onion, chopped	1 tbsp (15 ml)
Chervil	1 pinch
Oregano	1 pinch
Tarragon	1 pinch
Chives, to taste	

For one serving:

Carbohydrates:	5 g = 1 unit
Fat:	17 g = 3.5 units
Proteins:	21 g
Calories:	268

❖

Beef Stroganov

In a non-stick pan, brown the onion first, then the meat. Drain. Add mushrooms, broth, salt, basil, nutmeg and pepper. Bring to a boil and let simmer on medium heat for 30 minutes. Before serving, mix yogurt with lemon juice and stir into the meat mixture. Garnish with parsley. Makes 2 servings.

Beef in strips lean cut	6 oz (180 g)
Onion, minced	1 cup (250 ml)
Fresh mushrooms, sliced	1 cup (250 ml)
Chicken broth	⅔ cup (160 ml)
Plain yogurt, 2 %	½ cup (125 ml)
Lemon juice	1 tsp (5 ml)
Basil	¼ tsp (1 ml)
Nutmeg	¼ tsp (1 ml)
Parsley, chopped	1 tbsp (15 ml)
Salt and black pepper, to taste	

For one serving:

Carbohydrates:	20 g = 5 units
Fat:	12 g = 2.5 units
Proteins:	31 g
Calories:	305

❖

Swedish Meatballs

In a small bowl, combine ground beef with shallot, mustard, thyme and pepper. Shape into small meatballs and cook slightly in non-stick pan until browned. Add mushrooms and cook a few more minutes. Then add water and beef consommé. Cook on medium heat for 8 to 10 minutes. Sprinkle with parsley before serving. Makes 1 serving.

Beef, lean ground	4 oz (120 g)
Shallot, chopped	2 tbsp (30 ml)
Fresh mushrooms, sliced	4
Consommé (beef), powder	1 tps (5 ml)
Mustard	¼ tsp (1 ml)
Water	½ cup (125 ml)
Parsley, chopped	
Thyme and black pepper	1 pinch

For one serving:
Carbohydrates: 6 g = 1.5 units
Fat: 18 g = 3.5 units
Proteins: 24 g
Calories: 282

❖

Chinese Meatballs

Combine meat, salt, onion powder, pepper and mix. Shape into 4 meatballs. Bake at 350 °F/180 °C for 10 minutes. Place meatballs in a baking dish, add vegetables and broth. Bake at 450 °F/230 °C for 1 hour or until vegetables are tender. Makes 2 servings.

Beef, lean ground	8 oz (240 g)
Broth (beef)	2 tsp (10 ml)
Bean sprouts	2 cups (500 ml)
Green pepper, chopped	½ cup (125 ml)
Onion, minced	1 tsp (5 ml)
Water	2 cups (500 ml)
Black pepper and salt	

For one serving:

Carbohydrates:	11 g = 3 units
Fat:	21 g = 4 units
Proteins:	30 g
Calories:	351

❖

Beef Brochette

In a bowl, combine beef cubes, soy sauce and wine vinegar. Mix well and put in the refrigerator. Marinate at least 2 hours. Drain the meat. Cut the tomato and green pepper in wedges. On a skewer, thread beef cubes alternating with tomato and green pepper. Heat oven to broil and grill the brochette for 12 to 15 minutes. Turn the brochette throughout the cooking. Add salt and pepper when cooked. Makes 1 serving.

Beef, cubed lean cut	4 oz (120 g)
Soy sauce, sugar free	2 tbsp (30 ml)
Wine vinegar	2 tbsp (30 ml)
Tomato, fresh	1
Green pepper	½ cup (125 ml)
Oregano, dry	1 tsp (5 ml)
Salt and black pepper, to taste	

For one serving:

Carbohydrates:	16 g =	4 units
Fat:	9 g =	2 units
Proteins:	30 g	
Calories:	259	

❖

Meatball Brochettes

Combine meat, onion, herbs and pepper. Mix well and shape into meatballs. On a skewer, thread meatballs, alternating with vegetables. Brush with Worcestershire sauce. Microwave, uncovered, at full power for 2 minutes and serve. Makes 1 serving.

Beef, lean ground	4 oz (120 g)
Green pepper, pieces	½ cup (125 ml)
Fresh mushrooms	3 cups (750 ml)
Tomato wedges	2
Onion, chopped	1 tbsp (15 ml)
Oregano	1 pinch
Worcestershire sauce	1 tsp (5 ml)
Garlic, chopped	1 tsp (5 ml)
Black pepper, to taste	

For one serving:

Carbohydrates:	33 g = 8 units
Fat:	15 g = 3 units
Proteins:	31 g
Calories:	407

❖

Tarragon Patty

Combine all ingredients and shape into a patty. Cook the patty in a non-stick pan. Makes 1 serving.

Beef, lean ground	4 oz (120 g)
Tarragon	½ tsp (2 ml)
Shallot, chopped	2
Garlic, minced	1 clove
Salt and black pepper, to taste	

For one serving:

Carbohydrates:	2 g = 0.5 unit
Fat:	17 g = 2.5 units
Proteins:	21 g
Calories:	251

❖

Meatballs with Green Pepper

Combine the meat, salt, garlic and pepper. Mix well and shape into meatballs (4). Grill at 425 °C/220 °C for 15 minutes. Then place the meatballs in a casserole, add green and red pepper and onion slices. Add broth, cover. Heat on medium for 15 minutes or until vegetables are tender. Makes 2 servings.

Beef, lean ground	8 oz (240 g)
Green pepper, chopped	½ cup (125 ml)
Red pepper, chopped	½ cup (125 ml)
Onion, sliced	½ cup (125 ml)
Consommé (beef)	½ tsp (2 ml)
Garlic, chopped	1 clove
Water	½ cup (125ml)
Salt and black pepper	

For one serving:

Carbohydrates:	12 g = 3 units
Fat:	18 g = 3.5 units
Proteins:	23 g
Calories:	295

Beef and Tomato Stew

In a non-stick pan brown the beef cubes. Drain and put in a baking dish. Add all other ingredients. Cover. Bake at 300 °F/150 °C for 2 ½ hours. Before serving, garnish with parsley. Makes 4 servings.

Beef, cubed lean cut	1 lb (454 g)
Onion wedges	2
Carrot, sliced	4
Fresh celery, sliced	2 stalks
Fresh mushrooms	12
Tomatoes, peeled and cut	1 cup (250 ml)
Consommé (beef)	1 ½ cup (375 ml)
Basil	¼ tsp (1 ml)
Garlic, chopped	1 clove
Thyme	¼ tsp (1 ml)
Parsley, chopped	1 tbsp (15 ml)
Salt, to taste	
Black pepper, to taste	

For one serving:

Carbohydrates:	15 g = 4 units
Fat:	9 g = 2 units
Proteins:	29 g
Calories:	252

❖

Chop Suey

Cook the green pepper, celery and onion in half of the beef broth on low heat for 10 minutes. In a non-stick pan, brown the beef cubes and then combine all ingredients, cover. Cook on low heat for 10 minutes. Makes 2 servings.

Green pepper, chopped	½ cup (125 ml)
Fresh celery, sliced	1 cup (250 ml)
Onion, minced	¼ cup (60 ml)
Consommé (beef)	2 cups (500 ml)
Beef, cubed	8 oz (240 g)
Bean sprouts	2 cups (500 ml)
Soy sauce, sugar free	2 tbsp (30 ml)
Garlic clove, minced	1
Ginger, minced	1 tbsp (15 ml)

For one serving:

Carbohydrates:	18 g= 4.5 units
Fat:	9 g = 2 units
Proteins:	35 g
Calories:	287

❖

Beef Chow Mein

Combine meat and onion and brown in a non-stick skillet. Drain fat, add zucchini. Cover and cook for a few minutes. Add the remaining ingredients. Keep the dish covered while cooking over low heat for 5 to 10 minutes. Makes 2 servings.

Note: You can use chicken instead of beef.

Beef, lean ground	8 oz (240 g)
Onion, chopped	2 tbsp (30 ml)
Fresh celery, chopped	¼ cup (60 ml)
Bean sprouts	½ cup (125 ml)
Fresh mushrooms, sliced	½ cup (125 ml)
Zucchini, sliced	½ cup (125 ml)
Garlic, minced	1 tsp (5 ml)
Ginger, minced	2 tsp (10 ml)

For one serving:

Carbohydrates:	9 g = 2 units
Fat:	18 g = 3.5 units
Proteins:	24 g
Calories:	283

❖

Parisian Patties

Shape meat into 4 patties and add pepper. Place garlic, mushrooms, basil and parsley into a microwave-safe dish. Microwave covered at full power for 3 minutes. Add tomatoes and patties. Microwave covered at full power for 4 minutes. Remove patties, add tomato paste and mustard to thicken the sauce. Microwave, covered, at full power for 1 minute. Top patties with mushroom sauce. Makes 2 servings.

Beef, lean ground	8 oz (240 g)
Garlic clove, chopped	1 clove
Fresh mushrooms, sliced	1 cup (250 ml)
Basil	1 tsp (5 ml)
Parsley	1 tsp (5 ml)
Italian Tomatoes	1 cup (250 ml)
Tomato paste	2 tsp (10 ml)
Dijon mustard	1 tsp (5 ml)
Salt and black pepper	1 pinch

For one serving:	
Carbohydrates:	10 g = 2 units
Fat:	18 g = 3.5 units
Proteins:	25 g
Calories:	330

❖

Italian Beef Cubes

Combine beef broth with tomatoes, shallot and seasonings.
Add beef cubes and simmer, uncovered, on medium heat for
45 minutes. Makes 2 servings.

Beef, cubed lean cut	8 oz (240 g)
Broth (beef)	3 cups (750 ml)
Tomatoes, peeled and sliced	2
Shallot, chopped	2 tbsp (30 ml)
Oregano	¼ tsp (1 ml)
Basil	¼ tsp (1 ml)
Salt and black pepper, to taste	

For one serving:
Carbohydrates: 6 g = 1.5 units
Fat: 9 g = 2 units
Proteins: 30 g
Calories: 231

❖

Beef Sandwich

Mince the meat and mix with the low-calorie mayonnaise, the mustard and the shallots. Cut the slice of bread in two. Place the lettuce leaf on half slice, spread the meat mixture and cover with the other half of the slice. Makes 1 serving.

Beef, lean roast	4 oz (120 g)
Mayonnaise, light	1 tbsp (15 ml)
Shallot, chopped	1 tbsp (15 ml)
Lettuce leaf	
Sliced bread (whole wheat)	1 slice
Mustard (Dijon)	1 tsp (5 ml)
Salt and pepper	1 pinch

For one serving:

Carbohydrates: 15 g = 4 units
Fat: 14 g = 3 units
Proteins: 30 g
Calories: 308

❖

Goulash

Coat beef cubes with paprika. Place meat in baking dish and add onion. Microwave at full power for 1 ½ minute. Add all others ingredients. Cover and microwave at medium-high (70 %) for 6 minutes. Let stand 5 minutes and garnish with parsley. Makes 1 serving.

Beef, cubed lean cut	4 oz (120 g)
Onion, chopped	1 tbsp (15 ml)
Tomato paste	1 tbsp (15 ml)
Water	¾ cup (180 ml)
Consommé (onion)	2 tbsp (30 ml)
Paprika	1 pinch
Bay leaf	1
Thyme	½ tsp (2 ml)
Parsley, chopped	1 bouquet

For one serving:

Carbohydrates:	4 g = 1 unit
Fat:	7 g = 1.5 units
Proteins:	24 g
Calories:	178

❖

Italian Meat Loaf

In a big bowl, mix the meat with onion consommé, egg white, pepper, Italian seasoning and half the quantity of tomato sauce. Put the meat mixture on wax paper. Shape the meat mixture into a loaf shape. Put in a microwave-safe dish. Microwave, uncovered, at full power for 3 minutes. Microwave again 2 minutes at medium-high. Drain the juice from the loaf and cover with foil and let stand 5 minutes. When it's time to serve: top meatloaf with remaining tomato sauce and sprinkle with parmesan cheese. Microwave at full power for 40 seconds and serve. Makes 1 serving.

Beef, lean ground	6 oz (180 ml)
Mozzarella skimmed cheese, grated	2 tbsp (30 ml)
Consommé (onion)	2 tsp (10 ml)
Parmesan cheese, grated	1 tbsp (15 ml)
Egg, white	1
Tomato sauce	¼ cup (60 ml)
Oregano	½ tsp (2 ml)
Basil	½ tsp (2 ml)
Black pepper, to taste	

For one serving:
Carbohydrates: 6 g = 1.5 units
Fat: 33 g = 6.5 units
Proteins: 47 g
Calories: 517

❖

Seasoned Meat Loaf

Combine all ingredients and mix well. Put in a baking dish.
Bake at 375 °F/190 °C for 25 to 30 minutes or until the meat is
cooked. Drain juices from the loaf. Serve. Makes 2 servings.

Beef, lean ground	8 oz (240 g)
Tomato juice	½ cup (125 ml)
Green pepper, chopped	2 tbsp (30 ml)
Onion, chopped	2 tsp (10 ml)
Basil	⅛ tsp (0.5 ml)
Worcestershire sauce	¼ tsp (1 ml)
Salt and black pepper	

For one serving:

Carbohydrates:	4 g	= 1 unit
Fat:	17 g	= 3.5 units
Proteins:	22 g	
Calories:	260	

❖

Beef Strips

Put all ingredients, except the salt, in a microwave-safe dish and mix well. Cover and cook for 8 minutes on high. Let cool for 5 minutes. Lightly add salt and serve. Makes 1 servings.

Beef, strips lean cut	4 oz. (120 g)
Green pepper, cubed	1 tbsp (15 ml)
Onion, chopped	1 tbsp (15 ml)
White wine, dry	1 tsp (5 ml)
Tomato paste	½ tsp (2 ml)
Fresh mushrooms, sliced	3
Oregano	¼ tsp (1 ml)
Basil	¼ tsp (1 ml)
Cornstarch	¼ tsp (1 ml)
Worcestershire sauce	1 drop
Water	¼ cup (60 ml)
Salt and black pepper, to taste	

For one serving:

Carbohydrates:	5 g = 1 unit
Fat:	13 g = 3 units
Proteins:	32 g
Calories:	275

❖

Chicken Liver Brochette

Clean liver and marinate with vegetables in soy sauce. Refrigerate at least 30 minutes. On skewer, thread pieces of liver alternating with vegetables. Microwave, uncovered, at full power for 2 minutes. Makes 1 serving.

Livers (chicken)	4 oz (120 g)
Fresh mushrooms	3
Tomatoes (cherry)	3
Green pepper	3 pieces
Onion	3 pieces
Soy sauce, sugar free	2 tbsp (30 ml)

For one serving:

Carbohydrates:	20 g = 5 units
Fat:	5 g = 1 unit
Proteins:	26 g
Calories:	221

❖

Chicken Livers

Spray frying pan with Pam and add a small amount of water. Combine all ingredients and stir fry until livers are well done. Add more water if needed. Makes 1 serving.

Chicken livers	4 oz (120 g)
Fresh mushrooms, sliced	½ cup (125 ml)

SAUCE:

Tabasco sauce	4 drops
Onion, chopped	½ cup (125 ml)
Mustard, dry	1 pinch
Salt and black pepper, to taste	

For one serving:

Carbohydrates:	18 g = 4.5 units
Fat:	5 g = 1 unit
Proteins:	23 g
Calories:	204

❖

Sauted Chicken Livers

Cut the liver into thin strips. In a non-stick pan, cook the liver and add pepper, tomato paste, thyme, onion consommé and water. Cook 10 minutes on medium heat. Sprinkle with parsley and serve. Makes 1 serving.

Livers (chicken)	4 oz (120 g)
Tomato sauce	1 tbsp (15 ml)
Consommé (onion)	1 pouch
Water	½ cup (125 ml)
Parsley (optional), chopped	
Pepper green, sliced	½ cup (125 ml)
Thyme and black pepper	

For one serving:
Carbohydrates: 8 g = 2 units
Fat: 5 g = 1 unit
Proteins: 21 g
Calories: 159

❖

Calf's Liver with Basil

Place liver in baking dish. Add all others ingredients except salt. Microwave, covered, at full power for 2 minutes. Add little salt and pepper to taste. Sprinkle with parsley and serve. Makes 1 serving.

Livers (calf's)	4 oz (120 g)
Onion, minced	2 tbsp (30 ml)
Lemon juice	1 tbsp (15 ml)
Basil	½ tsp (2 ml)
Salt, black pepper and parsley, to taste	

For one serving:
Carbohydrates: 9 g = 2 units
Fat: 5 g = 1 unit
Proteins: 20 g
Calories: 164

Calf's Liver with White Leek

Place leek, consommé and water in baking dish. Cover and microwave at full power for 1 ½ minute. Add liver and cover. Microwave again at full power for 1 ½ minute. Remove the liver and add yogurt. Mix well and top liver with yogurt mixture. Serve hot. Makes 1 serving.

Liver (calf's)	4 oz (120 g)
Leek, white part	1
Consommé (chicken) (optional)	½ tsp (2 ml)
Plain yogurt, 0.1 %	1 tbsp (15 ml)
Water	¼ cup (60 ml)

For one serving:
Carbohydrates: 24 g = 6 units
Fat: 6 g = 1 unit
Proteins: 23 g
Calories: 236

❖

Liver with Fine Herbs

In a non-stick pan, cook mushrooms, carrots, green pepper and garlic for 5 minutes. Add the liver and cook until there is no longer pink inside. In a bowl, mix flour in 15 ml (1 tbsp) of chicken broth. Add broth mixture to vegetables and add the remaining ingredients, except parsley. Cook until the sauce thickens, stir often. Before serving, sprinkle with parsley. Makes 2 servings.

Fresh mushrooms, sliced	1 cup (250 ml)
Carrot, strips	½ cup (125 ml)
Green pepper, strips	½ cup (125 ml)
Garlic clove, chopped	1
Livers (calf's), strips	8 oz (240 g)
Chicken broth, fat free	½ cup (125 ml)
Flour	2 tsp (10 ml)
Tomatoes, peeled and crushed	1 cup (250 ml)
Rosemary, salt and black pepper, to taste	
Parsley (fresh), chopped, to taste	

For one serving:

Carbohydrates:	28 g = 7 units
Fat:	5 g = 1 unit
Proteins:	24 g
Calories:	250

❖

Calf's Liver with Vegetable

Microwave vegetables at full power for 2 minutes. Add all other ingredients and microwave at full power for 2 minutes. Let stand 4 minutes before serving. Makes 1 serving.

Livers (calf's)	4 oz (120 g)
Green pepper, minced	1 unit
Onion, minced	1 tbsp (15 ml)
Consommé (beef)	⅓ cup (80 ml)
Oregano	¼ tsp (1 ml)

For one serving:
Carbohydrates: 11 g = 3 units
Fat: 5 g = 1 unit
Proteins: 21 g
Calories: 175

❖

Peking Calf's Liver

Place vegetables in microwave-safe dish. Microwave, covered, at full power for 2 minutes. Add liver, soy sauce, parsley and pepper. Microwave, covered, at full power for 1 ½ minute. Serve. Makes 1 serving.

Livers (calf's)	4 oz (120 g)
Onion, chopped	1 tbsp (15 ml)
Green pepper, chopped	2 tbsp (30 ml)
Garlic clove, chopped	½ clove
Tomato wedges	1
Parsley (fresh)	1 tsp (5 ml)
Soy sauce, sugar free	½ tsp (2 ml)
Black pepper, to taste	

For one serving:
Carbohydrates: 13 g = 3 units
Fat: 5 g = 1 unit
Proteins: 22 g
Calories: 188

Calf's Liver with Green Pepper

Place calf's liver in a baking dish, and season it with onion powder, salt, pepper and green pepper. Broil liver for 8 to 10 minutes on both sides or until liver is cooked. Serve. Makes 1 serving.

Livers (calf's)	4 oz (120 g)
Green pepper, chopped	½ cup (125 ml)
Onion, minced	1 tsp (5 ml)
Garlic clove, chopped	1
Salt and black pepper, to taste	

For one serving:

Carbohydrates:	14 g = 3.5 units
Fat:	5 g = 1 unit
Proteins:	21 g
Calories:	189

❖

Pork Meatballs with Tomatoes

In a non-stick pan, cook onions and garlic until they are tender.
In a bowl, combine onions, garlic, meat, bread, yogurt, parsley,
salt, rosemary and pepper. Mix well and shape into meatballs
(8). In the oven, broil meatballs until they are browned. In a
non-stick pan, place meatballs, tomatoes and Worcestershire
sauce, stir. Cover and simmer for 30 minutes. Makes 2 servings.

Onion, chopped	½ cup (125 ml)
Garlic clove, chopped	1
Pork, lean ground	8 oz (240 g)
Plain yogurt, 2 %	2 tbsp (30 ml)
Sliced bread, cut into cubes	1 slice
Tomatoes, crushed (canned)	1 cup (250 ml)
Worcestershire sauce	1 tsp (5 ml)
Rosemary	¼ tsp (1 ml)
Parsley, chopped (fresh)	1 tbsp (15 ml)
Salt and black pepper, to taste	

For one serving:

Carbohydrates:	17 g = 4 units
Fat:	25 g = 5 units
Proteins:	23 g
Calories:	389

❖

Sweet–and–Sour Pork and Pineapple

In a non-stick pan, cook green pepper, carrot, garlic and shallots for 5 minutes or until vegetables are tender-crisp. Add meat, chicken broth, vinegar, soy sauce and brown sugar. Stir and bring to a boil. Reduce heat and simmer for 5 minutes. In a small bowl, mix cornstarch with water. Add cornstarch mixture and pineapple in pan. Cook until mixture thickens. Stir often. Makes 2 servings.

Green pepper, in thin strips	½ cup (125 ml)
Carrot, thinly sliced	¼ cup (60 ml)
Shallot, chopped	¼ cup (60 ml)
Garlic clove, chopped	2
Pork, cubed, cooked	6 oz (180 g)
Chicken broth	½ cup (125 ml)
Wine vinegar	2 tsp (10 ml)
Soy sauce, sugar free	2 tsp (10 ml)
Water	1 tbsp (15 ml)
Cornstarch	2 tsp (10 ml)
Pineapple chunks	½ cup (125 ml)

For one serving:

Carbohydrates:	24 g = 6 units
Fat:	18 g = 3.5 units
Proteins:	24 g
Calories:	341

❖

Pineapple Pork

In a non-stick pan, brown pork and onions on low heat for 10 minutes. Then add seasonings, water and pineapple juice. Cover and simmer for 30 minutes. Lastly, arrange the pineapple slices, green pepper and cornstarch dissolved in cold water, over the pork. Cook until it thickens (10 minutes). Makes 2 servings.

Pork, cubed	8 oz (240 g)
Onion, chopped	¼ cup (60 ml)
Vinegar	1 tbsp (15 ml)
Soy sauce, sugar free	1 tbsp (15 ml)
Water	¼ cup (60 ml)
Pineapple juice, unsweetened	¼ cup (60 ml)
Pineapple, sliced	3
Green pepper, sliced	1
Cornstarch	2 tsp (10 ml)
Water, cold	1 tbsp (15 ml)
Salt and black pepper, to taste	

For one serving:
Carbohydrates: 28 g = 7 units
Fat: 8 g = 1.5 units
Proteins: 24 g
Calories: 270

❖

Pork with Onion and Apples

Preheat oven grill. Spread mustard on both sides of pork chop and place on pan broiler. Broil pork chop, turn to broil on both sides. In a non-stick pan, brown onions and apple slices. Reduce heat and sprinkle with savory. Cover and let cook until apples are tender, stirring occasionally. Put pork chop in a serving dish top with apple sauce and garnish with parsley. Makes 1 serving.

Pork chop	4 oz (120 g)
Mustard, spicy	1 tsp (5 ml)
Apple (peeled), sliced	1
Onion, sliced	¼ cup (60 ml)
Savory (ground)	¼ tsp (1 ml)
Parsley	
Butter or olive oil	½ tsp (2 ml)

For one serving:
Carbohydrates: 24 g = 6 units
Fat: 6 g = 1 unit
Proteins: 25 g
Calories: 253

❖

Pork "Fried" Rice

In a non-stick pan, heat oil and reheat rice and soy sauce stirring often. Add shallots, brown them until tender. Add meat and reheat until heated through. Gradually add egg and cook until egg thickens. Serve immediately. Makes 2 servings.

Vegetable oil	1 tsp (5 ml)
Rice (long grain), cooked	1 cup (250 ml)
Soy sauce, sugar free	1 tbsp (15 ml)
Shallot, chopped	¼ cup (60 ml)
Pork, cubed and cooked	6 oz (180 g)
Egg, beaten	1

For one serving:

Carbohydrates:	32 g = 8 units
Fat:	15 g = 5 units
Proteins:	28 g
Calories:	375

❖

Ham Rolls

In a non-stick pan, cook onion, add mushrooms and cook for 2 minutes. Remove from heat. Spoon vegetable onto each ham slice. Arrange broccoli stalk over vegetables. Roll ham slices and put in baking dish. SAUCE: Melt butter then add water and flour (cook on medium heat). Pour milk gradually, heat until it thickens (while stirring). Add seasonings and grated cheese. Cook on low heat until the cheese melts. Top each roll with this sauce. Cover and bake at 350 °F/180 °C for 20 minutes, uncover and continue cooking for 5 more minutes. Makes 2 servings.

Onion, chopped	¼ cup (60 ml)
Fresh mushrooms, chopped	1 cup (250 ml)
Ham, cooked	6 slices (180 g)
Broccoli, frozen	10 oz (300 g)
SAUCE:	
Butter	1 tsp (5 ml)
Flour	2 tsp (10 ml)
2 % partially skim milk	½tsp (5 ml)
Black pepper, to taste	
Low fat cheese, grated	¼ cup (60 ml)
Curry	½ tsp (2 ml)
Salt	

For one serving:
Carbohydrates: 26 g = 6.5 units
Fat: 14 g = 3 units
Proteins: 48 g
Calories: 420

Veal Steak with Paprika

In a non-stick pan, slightly cook the veal steak. Then add the onion and tomatoes and sprinkle with paprika. Add a little salt and pepper. Add water, cover and simmer on low heat for 10 minutes. Serve hot. Makes 1 serving.

Veal, sliced	4 oz (120 g)
Tomatoes, cubed	1 tomato
Onion, thinly chopped	1
Paprika, to taste	
Water	2 tbsp (30 ml)
Salt, to taste	
Black pepper, to taste	

For one serving:
Carbohydrates: 11 g = 3 units
Fat: 3 g = 0.5 unit
Proteins: 25 g
Calories: 170

❖

Veal Blanquette

Place veal, onion, parsley, water and bay leaf in microwave-safe dish. Microwave at medium-low (50 %) for 15 minutes. Let stand 5 minutes. Microwave mushrooms at full power for 1 minute. Remove parsley branch and bay leaf from meat and add mushrooms. Add salt, pepper and yogurt to meat and mix well. Sprinkle with parsley and serve. Makes 1 serving.

Veal, cubed	4 oz (120 g)
Onion, sliced	½
Parsley, branch	1
Fresh mushrooms, minced	3
Bay leaf	1
Plain yogurt, 2 %	1 tbsp (15 ml)
Water	½ cup (125 ml)
Parsley, chopped	1 tsp (5 ml)
Salt and black pepper, to taste	

For one serving:

Carbohydrates:	9 g = 2 units
Fat:	3 g = 0.5 unit
Proteins:	25 g
Calories:	170

❖

Indian Meatballs

In a bowl, combine ground veal with onion, garlic, curry, cinnamon and cayenne pepper. Shape into small meatballs. In a non-stick pan, brown the meatballs, add water and onion consommé. Cook on medium heat for 8 minutes. Serve hot. Garnish with a lemon slice. Makes 1 serving.

Veal, chopped	4 oz (120 g)
Onion, chopped	1 tbsp (15 ml)
Garlic clove, chopped	1 clove
Curry	¼ tsp (1 ml)
Cinnamon	¼ tsp (1 ml)
Cayenne pepper	¼ tsp (1 ml)
Water	½ cup (125 ml)
Consommé (onion)	½ tsp (2 ml)
Cauliflower, sliced	½ cup (125 ml)
Spinach, chopped	½ cup (125 ml)
Lemon, sliced	1

For one serving:

Carbohydrates:	5 g = 1 unit
Fat:	5 g = 1 unit
Proteins:	23 g
Calories:	156

❖

Veal Brochette

In a bowl, mix the wine vinegar, Worcestershire sauce and add seasonings. Cut veal into 4 cubes and marinate the meat 2 hours or more. When meat is marinated, on a skewer, thread pieces of veal alternating with vegetables. Microwave at full power for 2 minutes. Turn skewer over while cooking. Let stand 3 minutes before serving. Makes 1 serving.

Veal fillet	4 oz (120 g)
Green pepper, chunks	½ cup (125 ml)
Tomatoes, wedges	2
Zucchini, sliced	3
Fresh mushrooms	3
Wine vinegar	2 tbsp (30 ml)
Worcestershire sauce	1 tbsp (15 ml)
Peppercorns, oregano and chervil, to taste	

For one serving:
Carbohydrates:	20 g = 5 units
Fat:	4 g = 1 unit
Proteins:	29 g
Calories:	221

❖

Veal Meatballs with Chervil

Combine all ingredients. Shape the meat into one patty. Put in the oven and cook each side for 7 minutes at 350 °F/180 °C. Makes 1 serving.

Veal, lean (minced)	4 oz (120 g)
Chervil	½ tsp (2 ml)
Shallot, chopped	1 tsp (5 ml)
Garlic powder	1 clove
Salt and pepper, to taste	

For one serving:
Carbohydrates: 1 g
Fat: 3 g = 0.5 unit
Proteins: 23 g
Calories: 131

❖

Veal Cutlet Bonne-Femme

Season the veal cutlets and put in a baking dish. Add vegetables, alternating potato slices and onion slices ending with potatoes. Then mix mustard, curry powder and chicken broth. Pour broth mixture over cutlets and vegetables. Sprinkle with paprika. Cover and bake at 350 °F/180 °C about 1 hour. Makes 2 servings.

Veal (cutlets)	2 of 4 oz (120 g)
Onion, sliced	½ cup (125 ml)
Potato, sliced and peeled	2
Dijon mustard	¼ tsp (1 ml)
Curry	1 pinch
Chicken broth, fat free	¾ cup (180 ml)
Paprika, to taste	
Salt	1 tsp (5 ml)
Black pepper	½ tsp (2 ml)

For one serving:

Carbohydrates:	24 g = 6 units
Fat:	4 g = 1 unit
Proteins:	28 g
Calories:	243

❖

Veal Croquette

Mix meat with onion and herbs. Shape into patties (2). Add salt and pepper. Place mushrooms and green pepper in baking dish. Cover and microwave at full power for 2 minutes. Add patties and the other ingredients to the vegetables. Dissolve cornstarch in water, add soy sauce and rosemary. Cover and microwave at full power for 2 minutes. Let stand 2 or 3 minutes. Serve. Makes 1 serving.

Veal, lean ground	4 oz (120 g)
Onion, chopped	1 tbsp (15 ml)
Green pepper, minced	½ cup (125 ml)
Parsley, chopped	1 tsp (5 ml)
Broth (chicken)	¼ tsp (1 ml)
Water	¼ cup (60 ml)
Soy sauce, sugar free	½ tsp (2 ml)
Fresh mushrooms, minced	4
Cornstarch	¼ tsp (1 ml)
Rosemary	¼ tsp (1 ml)
Salt and black pepper, to taste	

For one serving:

Carbohydrates:	8 g = 2 units
Fat:	8 g = 1.5 units
Proteins:	25 g
Calories:	208

❖

Hungarian Veal Cutlets

Brown cutlets on both sides and place them in baking dish. Add onion rings and pour in chicken broth. Add paprika, salt and pepper. Cover. Bake at 375 °F/190 °F for 15 minutes or until cutlets are tender. Remove the cover. Raise oven temperature to 500 °F/260 °C for 5 minutes or until pan juices have evaporated. Add yogurt and cook until heated through. Do not boil. Makes 2 servings.

Veal (cutlets)	2 of 4 oz (120 g)
Onion, sliced	¼ cup (60 ml)
Chicken broth	3 tbsp (45 ml)
Plain yogurt, 2 %	⅓ cup (80 ml)
Paprika	½ tsp (2 ml)
Salt and black pepper, to taste	

For one serving:

Carbohydrates:	5 g = 1 unit
Fat:	3 g = 0.5 unit
Proteins:	28 g
Calories:	164

❖

Paprika Veal Cutlet

Place onion in baking dish and microwave at full power for 2 minutes. Sprinkle paprika on both sides of veal cutlet and place veal on cooked onion. Microwave at full power for 1 minute and let stand 3 minutes. Before serving, mix yogurt with pan juices and spread this sauce over the meat. Makes 1 serving.

Onion, minced	1 tbsp (15 ml)
Plain yogurt, 2 %	1 tsp (5 ml)
Veal cutlet	4 oz (120 g)
Paprika, salt and black pepper, to taste	

For one serving:

Carbohydrates:	21 g = 5 units
Fat:	5 g = 1 unit
Proteins:	29 g
Calories:	250

❖

Veal Cutlet au Gratin

Place veal cutlet in a baking dish. Add onion consommé and water. Sprinkle with tarragon and grated cheese. Bake at 450 °F/230 °C for 15 minutes. Serve. Makes 1 serving.

Veal (cutlet)	4 oz (120 g)
Consommé (onion), fat free	¼ tsp (1 ml)
Water	2 tbsp (30 ml)
Tarragon, to taste	
Cheese, grated	2 tbsp (30 ml)

For one serving:

Carbohydrates:	2 g = 0.5 unit
Fat:	4 g = 1 unit
Proteins:	32 g
Calories:	182

Veal Cutlet Parmesan

Place veal in microwave-safe dish. Add cheese, spices and to-mato sauce. Microwave at full power for 1 ½ minute. Serve hot. Makes 1 serving.

Veal cutlet	4 oz (120 g)
Tomato sauce	2 tbsp (30 ml)
Oregano	¼ tsp (1 ml)
Basil	¼ tsp (1 ml)
Parmesan cheese, grated	3 tbsp (45 ml)
Chili powder	¼ tsp (1 ml)

For one serving:
Carbohydrates: 6 g = 1.5 units
Fat: 10 g = 2 units
Proteins: 31 g
Calories: 239

❖

Spicy Veal Cutlet

Season veal cutlet with salt, pepper and lemon juice. Then brown the meat in a non-stick pan. Remove meat. Cook onions until tender, then add veal, rosemary, tabasco and lemon slices. Cook at a medium heat for 8 to 10 minutes. Garnish with parsley. Makes 2 servings.

Veal (cutlets)	2 of 4 oz (120 g)
Lemon juice	1 tbsp (15 ml)
Onion, chopped	1 cup (15 ml)
Rosemary	1 tsp (5 ml)
Tabasco sauce	$\frac{1}{4}$ tsp (1 ml)
Lemon, sliced	$\frac{1}{2}$
Parsley, chopped, to taste	
Salt and black pepper	1 pinch

For one serving:
Carbohydrates: 10 g = 2.5 units
Fat: 2 g = 0.5 unit
Proteins: 24 g
Calories: 170

❖

Veal Patties

In a non-stick pan, brown onions and garlic until onions are tender. Place cooked onions in bowl, add veal, half of bread crumbs, egg, parsley, lemon juice and seasonings. Mix well and shape into patties (2). Roll in remaining bread crumbs. In the non-stick pan, melt butter and cook patties on medium heat until patties are browned on both sides. Place veal patties in serving dish and keep warm. Sprinkle flour in pan juice and stir. Gradually add chicken broth, bring to a boil, stirring often. Reduce heat and simmer until it thickens. Top patties with sauce. Makes 2 servings.

Veal chopped (ground)	8 oz (240 g)
Onion, chopped	½ cup (125 ml)
Garlic clove, chopped	1
Bread crumbs	⅓ cup (80 ml)
Egg	1
Parsley, chopped	1 tbsp (15 ml)
Lemon juice	1 tbsp (15 ml)
Butter	1 tsp (5 ml)
Nutmeg	¼ tsp (1 ml)
Flour	1 tsp (5 ml)
Chicken broth, fat free	¾ cup (180 ml)
Salt	½ tsp (2 ml)
Black pepper, to taste	

For one serving:

Carbohydrates:	17 g = 4 units
Fat:	18 g = 3.5 units
Proteins:	28 g
Calories:	334

❖

Indian Veal

In bowl, place meat, add half the onion, half the parsley and basil, curry and pepper. Mix well and shape into 8 meatballs. In a microwave-safe dish, place chicken broth, remaining onion, mushrooms, parsley, basil, Worcestershire sauce and pepper. Microwave, covered, at full power for 5 minutes or until it boils. Place meatballs in the boiling liquid. Microwave, covered, at full power for 10 minutes. Add tomato paste, mustard and re-maining curry. Microwave covered at full power for 3 more minutes. Makes 2 servings.

Veal, lean ground	8 oz (240 g)
Onion, chopped	½ cup (125 ml)
Fresh mushrooms, sliced	½ cup (125 ml)
Worcestershire sauce	½ tsp (2 ml)
Basil	½ tsp (2 ml)
Curry	1 tsp (5 ml)
Chicken broth	1 cup (250 ml)
Tomato paste	½ tbsp (7 ml)
Black pepper	1 pinch
Dijon mustard	1 tsp (5 ml)
Parsley	2 tbsp (30 ml)

For one serving:

Carbohydrates:	8 g	= 2 units
Fat:	9 g	= 2 units
Proteins:	26 g	
Calories:	225	

❖

Veal with Carrots

Brown veal in a non-stick pan. Add carrot slices, onion consommé and water. Sprinkle with thyme and pepper. Cook on low heat for 10 minutes. Before serving, sprinkle with parsley. Makes 1 serving.

Veal, thin strips	4 oz (120 g)
Carrot, sliced	½ cup (125 ml)
Consommé (onion)	2 tsp (10 ml)
Water	¾ cup (180 ml)
Thyme	½ tsp (2 ml)
Parsley, chopped, to taste	
Black pepper, to taste	

For one serving:
Carbohydrates:	12 g = 3 units
Fat:	2 g = 0.5 unit
Proteins:	25 g
Calories:	167

❖

Veal with Fine Herbs

In a non-stick pan, slightly cook the veal until browned. First add salt and pepper, then the onions and mushrooms. Sprinkle with tarragon and chervil. Cook until onion is brown. Add water and yogurt and let simmer on low heat for 10 minutes. Makes 1 serving.

Veal, sliced	4 oz (120 g)
Fresh mushrooms, minced	½ cup (125 ml)
Plain yogurt, 2 %	2 tbsp (30 ml)
Water	¼ cup (60 ml)
Onion, minced	1 tbsp (15 ml)
Tarragon, to taste	
Chervil, to taste	
Salt, to taste	
Black pepper, to taste	

For one serving:

Carbohydrates:	6 g = 1.5 units
Fat:	3 g = 0.5 unit
Proteins:	28 g
Calories:	159

❖

Braised Veal with Mushrooms

Over oven grill, brown veal cutlet on both sides. In a non-stick pan, cook onion and garlic until tender. Add veal and all other ingredients. Let simmer on low heat for 10-15 minutes or until the veal is tender. Makes 1 serving.

Veal cutlet	4 oz (120 g)
Onion slices	¼ cup (60 ml)
Garlic clove, half	1
Fresh mushrooms, sliced	¼ cup (60 ml)
Lemon juice	1 tsp (5 ml)
Water	2 tsp (10 ml)
Oregano	¼ tsp (1 ml)
Parsley, chopped	1 tsp (5 ml)
Salt, to taste	

For one serving:

Carbohydrates:	8 g = 2 units	
Fat:	2 g = 0.5 unit	
Proteins:	26 g	
Calories:	155	

❖

Asparagus Chicken

Add yogurt to chicken cubes. In a non-stick pan, place asparagus and top with chicken and yogurt. Season with basil and pepper. Sprinkle with grated cheese and bake at 400 °F/200 °C for 20 minutes. Makes 1 serving.

Chicken, cubed (cooked)	4 oz (120 g)
Plain yogurt, 2 %	2 tbsp (30 ml)
Asparagus (canned)	½ cup (125 ml)
Basil	
Cheese, grated	3 tbsp (45 ml)
Black pepper	

For one serving:
Carbohydrates: 6 g = 1.5 units
Fat: 31 g = 6 units
Proteins: 40 g
Calories: 466

❖

Tomato Turkey Meatballs

MEATBALLS:

Preheat your oven at 350 °F/180 °C. Combine ground turkey, rice, onion, parsley, salt, marjoram, thyme and pepper. Shape into meatballs (6) and put in a non-stick pan.

SAUCE:

In a bowl, combine the remaining ingredients: tomato sauce, chicken broth and garlic. Top meatballs with the sauce and bake at 350 °F/180 °C for 45 minutes, stirring once. Makes 2 servings.

Turkey, lean ground	8 oz (240 g)
Rice, uncooked	¼ cup (60 ml)
Onion, chopped	¼ cup (60 ml)
Parsley, chopped	2 tbsp (30 ml)
Marjoram	1 pinch
Thyme	1 pinch
Salt and black pepper	

SAUCE:

Tomato sauce	1 cup (250 ml)
Chicken broth	½ cup (125 ml)
Garlic clove, chopped	½ tsp (2 ml)

For one serving:
Carbohydrates: 32 g = 8 units
Fat: 10 g = 2 units
Proteins: 25 g
Calories: 318

❖

Teriyaki Chicken Brochette

Place chicken cubes, pineapple chunks, soy sauce, vegetables and ginger in bowl. Let marinate at least 2 hours in refrigerator. On skewer, thread chicken alternating with vegetables and pineapple chunks. Microwave at full power for 3 ½ minutes. Makes 1 serving.

Chicken, cubed	4 oz (120 g)
Pineapple chunks	½ cup (125 ml)
Soy sauce, sugar free	1 tbsp (15 ml)
Garlic clove, chopped	1
Fresh mushrooms	3
Green pepper wedges	½ cup (125 ml)
Ginger fresh	2 slices

For one serving:
Carbohydrates: 20 g = 5 units
Fat: 15 g = 3 units
Proteins: 28 g
Calories: 322

❖

Turkey Casserole

Cook all ingredients (except turkey and cheese), until the vegetables are tender. Add turkey and cook 5 minutes. Pour mixture
into casserole and sprinkle with cheese. Bake at 400 °F/205 °C
for 20 minutes. Makes 1 serving.

Turkey, cooked	3 oz (90 g)
Cheddar cheese, grated	1 oz (30 g)
Mustard, dry	1 pinch
Worcestershire sauce	½ tsp (2 ml)
Paprika	¼ tsp (1 ml)
Garlic, chopped	1 clove
Fresh mushrooms, sliced	½ cup (125 ml)
Green pepper, cubed	½ cup (125 ml)
Onion, chopped	1 tbsp (15 ml)

For one serving:
Carbohydrates: 14 g = 2.5 units
Fat: 12 g = 2.5 units
Proteins: 35 g
Calories: 304

❖

Oriental Turkey Casserole

Spray a small baking dish with Pam. Spread cheddar cheese on bottom. Top with vegetables, turkey and Swiss cheese. Bake at 325 °F/160 °C for 20 minutes. Makes 1 serving.

Turkey, cooked and cubed	2 oz (60 g)
Cheese Swiss, grated	¼ cup (60 ml)
Broccoli, cooked	¼ cup (60 ml)
Cauliflower, cooked	¼ cup (60 ml)
Cheddar cheese, grated	¼ cup (60 ml)

For one serving:
Carbohydrates: 8 g = 2 units
Fat: 41 g = 8 units
Proteins: 52 g
Calories: 595

❖

Chicken Chop Suey

Place all vegetables in microwave-safe dish. Microwave at full power for 3 minutes. Combine soy sauce with chicken and add to vegetables. Cover and microwave at full power for 1 minute. Serve. Makes 1 serving.

Chicken, cooked	3 oz (90 g)
Bean sprouts	1 cup (250 ml)
Green pepper, cubed	2 tbsp (30 ml)
Onion, chopped	1 tbsp (15 ml)
Fresh celery, sliced	1 tbsp (15 ml)
Soy sauce, sugar free	1 tbsp (15 ml)
Garlic, minced	½ tsp (2 ml)
Ginger, minced	1 tsp (5 ml)

For one serving:
Carbohydrates: 11 g = 3 units
Fat: 11 g = 2 units
Proteins: 24 g
Calories: 231

Chicken à l'Orange

Brown the chicken without skin in a non-stick skillet. Set aside. In the same pan, brown the onions until soft. Set the onions in casserole and add chicken, orange juice, broth, garlic, salt and pepper. Cover and put in oven at 325 °F (160 °C) for 1 hour. Garnish with parsley and orange rind. Makes 2 servings.

Chicken breasts   2 of 4 oz (120 g)
Onion rinds   ½ cup (125 ml)
Chicken broth, fat free   ½ cup (125 ml)
Garlic clove, mashed   1
Orange juice   ¼ cup (60 ml)
Salt   ¼ tsp (1 ml)
Black pepper and parsley, to taste

For one serving:
Carbohydrates: 9 g = 2 units
Fat: 2 g = 0.5 unit
Proteins: 27 g
Calories: 175

❖

Coq au Vin

Place water, consommé, onion, carrots, bay leaf and parsley in microwave – safe dish. Microwave, covered, at full power for 3 minutes. Add remaining ingredients except salt. Microwave, covered, at medium-high (70 %) for 8 minutes. Add salt and pepper and let stand 5 minutes before serving. Makes 1 serving.

Chicken	4 oz (120 g)
Onion, chopped	1 tbsp (15 ml)
Carrot, cubed	3 tbsp (45 ml)
Fresh mushrooms, minced	4
Consommé (beef)	½ tsp (2 ml)
Water	¼ cup (60 ml)
Parsley	2 branches
Bay leaf	1
Red wine	1 tbsp (15 ml)
Cornstarch	1 tsp (5 ml)
Salt and black pepper, to taste	

For one serving:

Carbohydrates:	11 g = 3 units
Fat:	2 g = 0.5 unit
Proteins:	27 g
Calories:	186

❖

Deviled Chicken Legs

Mix together oil, Worcestershire sauce, vinegar, onion, mustard, salt and pepper. Score the chicken legs with the point of a sharp knife and brush them with the sauce. Place them in a broiler pan, under the broiler for 8 to 10 minutes, basting frequently. Turn the chicken over, brush with more sauce and continue broiling for 8 to 10 minutes until done. Brush mushrooms with remaining sauce and add them to pan for the last 5 minutes. Garnish with parsley. Makes 4 servings.

Vegetable oil	1 tsp (5 ml)
Worcestershire sauce	1 tsp (5 ml)
Vinegar	1 tsp (5 ml)
Onion, finely chopped	1 tsp (5 ml)
Mustard (Dijon)	1 tsp (5 ml)
Chicken legs	4
Fresh mushrooms	4 cups (1 liter)
Parsley to garnish	
Salt and pepper, to taste	

For one serving:

Carbohydrates:	8 g = 2 units
Fat:	7 g = 1.5 units
Proteins:	30 g
Calories:	210

❖

Cantonese Chicken

Put chicken in saucepan without fat. Cook lightly until brown and keep warm. In microwave dish, place onion, garlic and parsley. Microwave at full power for 1 minute. Add beef consommé, water, tomato paste, soy sauce, tarragon and cornstarch. Mix well and add to chicken. Microwave at medium power for 3 minutes (70 %). Add mushrooms, pepper and salt. Microwave again at medium power for 3 ½ minutes. Let stand 5 minutes and garnish with parsley. Makes 1 serving.

Chicken	4 oz (120 g)
Onion, chopped	2 tbsp (30 ml)
Garlic clove, chopped	1
Parsley, chopped	½ tsp (2 ml)
Tarragon	¼ tsp (1 ml)
Consommé (beef)	½ tsp (2 ml)
Water	½ cup (125 ml)
Soy sauce, sugar free	¼ tsp (1 ml)
Fresh mushrooms, minced	4
Cornstarch	¼ tsp (1 ml)
Tomato paste	1 tsp (5 ml)
Salt, to taste	
Black pepper, to taste	

For one serving:

Carbohydrates: 7 g = 2 units
Fat: 2 g = 0.5 unit
Proteins: 27 g
Calories: 160

❖

Chicken à la Crème

In a small casserole, combine carrot, celery and chicken broth. Bring to a full boil and cook for 5 minutes. In a non-stick casserole dish, melt butter and add flour. Cook for 2 minutes stirring often. Remove from heat and add vegetables gradually. Return to heat and let simmer for 5 minutes, stirring often. Add chicken, milk and parsley. Let simmer for 5 minutes or until chicken is hot. Makes 2 servings.

Carrot, cubed	¼ cup (60 ml)
Fresh celery, cubed	¼ cup (60 ml)
Chicken broth	¾ cup (180 ml)
Butter	1 tsp (5 ml)
Flour	2 tsp (10 ml)
Chicken, cubed (cooked)	6 oz (180 g)
Skim milk, 2 %	¼ cup (60 ml)
Parsley (fresh), chopped	1 pinch
Black pepper	

For one serving:

Carbohydrates:	6 g = 1.5 units
Fat:	8 g = 1.5 units
Proteins:	22 g
Calories:	193

❖

Chicken à la Mode

Peel the skin and remove fat from the chicken breasts. Put them in a baking dish. Season with thyme, onion powder, salt and pepper. Add chicken broth and all other ingredients. Cover and bake at 400 °F/205 °C for 1 hour or until chicken has cooked. Makes 2 servings.

Chicken breasts	2 of 4 oz (120 g)
Chicken broth, fat free	¼ cup (60 ml)
Carrot, sliced	½ cup (125 ml)
Fresh celery, chopped	¼ cup (60 ml)
Cabbage, cut	½ cup (125 ml)
Onion, sliced	2 tbsp (30 ml)
Thyme	½ tsp (2 ml)
Onion powder	1 pinch
Salt, to taste	
Black pepper, to taste	

For one serving:

Carbohydrates:	11 g = 3 units
Fat:	2 g = 0.5 unit
Proteins:	27 g
Calories:	172

❖

Chicken Dijon

Remove skin from chicken. Sprinkle chicken lightly with salt and pepper. Mix mustard into yogurt. In another bowl, mix bread crumbs with thyme. Spread each piece of chicken with mustard mixture, then roll in bread-crumb mixture. Place chicken in a single layer on lightly greased baking sheet. Bake at 350 °F/180 °C for 35 to 40 minutes or until golden brown and meat is no longer pink. Makes 2 servings.

Chicken breast	2 of 4 oz (120 g)
Dijon mustard	2 tbsp (30 ml)
Plain yogurt, 2 %	¼ cup (60 ml)
Bread crumbs	¼ cup (60 ml)
Thyme	½ tsp (2 ml)
Salt and black pepper, to taste	

For one serving:

Carbohydrates:	8 g	= 2 units
Fat:	4 g	= 1 unit
Proteins:	28 g	
Calories:	184	

❖

Chicken Provençal

In a non-stick pan, cook the chicken until browned and add onion, garlic and cubed tomato. Add salt and pepper, basil and tomato juice. Let cook, uncovered on medium heat for 10 minutes. Serve warm. Makes 1 serving.

Chicken	4 oz (120 g)
Garlic clove, chopped	1
Onion, chopped	2 tbsp (30 ml)
Tomato, cubed	1
Tomato juice	½ cup (125 ml)
Basil, to taste	
Salt, to taste	
Black pepper, to taste	

For one serving:
Carbohydrates: 16 g = 4 units
Fat: 4 g = 1 unit
Proteins: 26 g
Calories: 195

❖

Spanish Chicken

Peel off chicken skin and fat. Wash and dry the breasts. Add salt and pepper. Put chicken in a non-stick pan and brown it. Remove chicken and set aside. In the same pan, brown onions and garlic before adding tomatoes and broth. Boil for about 2 minutes. Put in a casserole dish, add mushrooms and chicken. Cover and bake at 325 °F/160 °C for one hour. Garnish with parsley. Makes 2 servings.

Chicken breasts	2 of 4 oz (120 g)
Onion, minced	1 cup (250 ml)
Garlic clove, minced	2
Tomatoes, peeled	1 cup (250 ml)
Chicken broth, fat free	½ cup (125 ml)
Fresh mushrooms, sliced	½ cup (125 ml)
Parsley, chopped	

For one serving:

Carbohydrates:	18 g = 4.5 units
Fat:	2 g = 0.5 unit
Proteins:	28 g
Calories:	207

❖

Tarragon Chicken

Debone breast and put in a microwave-safe dish. Add water, tarragon and chicken consommé. Cover and microwave at medium-high (70 %) for 3 ½ minutes. Let stand 5 minutes before serving. Makes 1 serving.

Chicken breast	4 oz (120 g)
Tarragon	1 tbsp (15 ml)
Consommé (chicken)	½ tsp (2 ml)
Water	¼ cup (60 ml)

For one serving:	
Carbohydrates:	Trace amount
Fat:	3 g = 0.5 unit
Proteins:	28 g
Calories:	145

❖

Vinegar Chicken

Place all ingredients in a casserole dish (except salt and pepper). Cover and microwave at medium-high (70 %) for 3 ½ minutes. Let stand 3 minutes and add salt and pepper before serving. Makes 1 serving.

Chicken	4 oz (120 g)
Wine vinegar	1 tsp (5 ml)
Garlic clove, chopped	1
Tarragon	½ tsp (2 ml)
Tomato (canned)	1
Consommé, fat free (beef)	2 tbsp (30 ml)
Salt and black pepper	

For one serving:	
Carbohydrates:	8 g = 2 units
Fat:	4 g = 1 unit
Proteins:	24 g
Calories:	163

Chicken Alexandra

Place chicken without the skin, onion, water and onion con-sommé in a small casserole dish. Cover and microwave at medium-high (70 %) for 3 ½ minutes. Let stand 4 minutes. Mix asparagus purée well with yogurt and chicken broth. Add salt and pepper. Microwave asparagus tips at full power for 8 minutes. Place chicken in a plate and top with asparagus sauce. Garnish with asparagus tips. Makes 1 serving.

Chicken	3 oz (90 g)
Onion, minced	1 tbsp (15 ml)
Water	¼ cup (60 ml)
Consommé (onion)	¼ tsp (1 ml)
Asparagus tips	3 tips
Asparagus purée	⅓ cup (80 ml)
Plain yogurt, 2 %	1 tbsp (15 ml)
Pan juices	1 tbsp (15 ml)
Salt and pepper, to taste	

For one serving:

Carbohydrates:	13 g = 3 units
Fat:	4 g = 1 unit
Proteins:	28 g
Calories:	256

❖

Chicken with Orange

Place boned chicken in microwave-safe dish. Add curry powder, orange juice, onion rings and pepper. Microwave covered for 6 minutes. Let stand 5 minutes, meanwhile add the orange wedges. Dress the chicken in a serving dish and serve. Makes 1 serving.

Chicken, boned	4 oz (120 g)
Orange juice	2 tbsp (30 ml)
Curry powder	½ tsp (2 ml)
Orange wedge	1
Onion	2 slices
Pepper	1 pinch

For one serving:

Carbohydrates: 24 g = 6 units
Fat: 4 g = 1 unit
Proteins: 24 g
Calories: 222

❖

Chicken Ascar

Pound (tenderize) the chicken until it is thin, separate into two pieces and season. Cook both sides of the breast, then place it in an oven dish. Add asparagus, crabmeat and cheese on top of the chicken. Cook at 350 °F/180 °C until the cheese has melted. Makes 2 servings.

Chicken breast (boneless)	4 oz (120 g)
Asparagus, cooked	6 tips
Canned crab	2 oz (60 g)
Cheese, sliced	2 oz (60 g)
Salt, to taste	
Black pepper, to taste	

For one serving:

Carbohydrates:	2 g = 0.5 unit
Fat:	11 g = 2 units
Proteins:	25 g
Calories:	213

❖

Chicken with Broccoli

Blanche broccoli, drain and put in glass dish. Cover broccoli with chicken slices.

SAUCE:

Combine broth, milk and seasonings and bring to a boil. Then mix cornstarch with water and add this mixture to the broth mixture. Cook until the sauce thickens. Add half of the parmesan cheese. Top chicken slices with sauce and sprinkle with grated parmesan cheese. Bake at 350 °F/180 °C for 15 minutes. Raise temperature to 450 °F/230 °C and cook a few more minutes until sauce has browned. Makes 2 servings.

Broccoli, in bunches	1 cup (250 ml)
Chicken, sliced and cooked	6 oz (180 g)
SAUCE:	
Chicken broth	1 ½ cup (375 ml)
2 % partially skimmed milk	⅓ cup (80 ml)
Cornstarch	2 tbsp (30 ml)
Water (cold)	2 tbsp (30 ml)
Parmesan cheese, grated	¼ cup (60 ml)

For one serving:

Carbohydrates: 18 g = 4.5 units
Fat: 18 g = 3.5 units
Proteins: 38 g
Calories: 380

❖

Chicken with Curry

In a microwave-safe dish, place chicken broth, celery, onion, garlic, curry, parsley, Worcestershire sauce and pepper. Microwave, covered, at full power (high) for 3 minutes or until it boils. Place skinned chicken breasts in boiling broth and microwave covered at full power for 12 minutes. Remove chicken from broth. Add tomato paste and mustard. Microwave, covered, at full power for 3 minutes. Serve chicken with sauce. Makes 2 servings.

Chicken breasts	2 of 4 oz (120 g)
Onion, chopped	1 cup (250 ml)
Fresh celery, chopped	½ cup (125 ml)
Garlic clove, chopped	1 clove
Worcestershire sauce	½ tsp (2 ml)
Curry	1 tbsp (15 ml)
Savory	½ tsp (2 ml)
Parsley	1 tsp (5 ml)
Chicken broth	1 cup (250 ml)
Tomato paste	2 tsp (10 ml)
Dijon mustard	2 tsp (10 ml)
Pepper	1 pinch

For one serving:

Carbohydrates:	15 g = 4 units
Fat:	4 g = 1 unit
Proteins:	34 g
Calories:	229

❖

Lemon Chicken

Remove fat from chicken and put in a casserole. Season, add lemon juice and chicken broth. Garnish with paprika. Cover and cook in oven at 350 °F/180 °C for 40 minutes. Serve each portion of 2 ½ ounces (75 g) with a lemon quarter and parsley. Makes 5 servings.

Chicken	3 lbs (1.4 kg)
Lemon juice (fresh)	¼ cup (60 ml)
Chicken broth, fat free	⅓ cup (80 ml)
Paprika	¼ tsp (1 ml)
Garlic clove, chopped	2
Lemon, wedges	5
Rosemary	½ tsp (2 ml)
Salt	¼ tsp (1 ml)

For one serving:

Carbohydrates:	2 g = 0.5 unit
Fat:	43 g = 8.5 units
Proteins:	47 g
Calories:	587

❖

Ginger Chicken with Peaches

In a glass bowl, mix teriyaki sauce, orange juice, garlic, ginger and chili powder. Add chicken. Stir. Cover and refrigerate for 1 hour at least. Remove chicken and keep marinade without garlic and ginger. In a non-stick pan, brown onions until tender. Add chicken and brown on each side. Mix cornstarch with marinade. Pour into pan. Bring to a boil, stirring often. Let simmer on low heat until sauce thickens. Add sliced peaches and snow peas. Stir and serve hot. Makes 2 servings.

Chicken strips	8 oz (240 g)
Teriyaki sauce	1 tbsp (15 ml)
Orange juice	1 tbsp (15 ml)
Garlic clove	1 tbsp (15 ml)
Ginger (fresh), grated	2 tsp (10 ml)
Chili powder	2 tsp (10 ml)
Onion, sliced	1 cup (250 ml)
Cornstarch	1 tsp (5 ml)
Peaches, sliced	1 ½ cup (375 ml)
Snow peas	1 cup (250 ml)

For one serving:

Carbohydrates:	54 g = 13.5 units
Fat:	2 g = 0.5 unit
Proteins:	36 g
Calories:	375

❖

Chicken with Green Pepper

In a non-stick pan, cook the onion on low heat until it is tender. Add green and red pepper, salt. Brown for 5 minutes and add chicken. Season and cover then let it simmer for 10 minutes. Serve. Makes 1 serving.

Chicken, cut, cooked	6 oz (180 g)
Onion, minced	½ cup (125 ml)
Green pepper, chopped	½ cup (125 ml)
Red pepper, chopped	½ cup (125 ml)
Salt	¼ tsp (1 ml)
Black pepper, to taste	

For one serving:

Carbohydrates:	17 g = 4 units
Fat:	5 g = 1 unit
Proteins:	36 g
Calories:	258

❖

Pressure Cooked Chicken

Place chicken in a 6-quart pressure cooker. Combine all ingredients and pour over chicken. Add broccoli, cauliflower or green beans. Do not fill cooker over ¾ full. Cook chicken 20 minutes after 10 pound pressure is reached. Remove cover. Skim fat off the broth and serve. Makes 6 servings.

Chicken, skinned	3 lbs (1.4 kg)
Paprika	½ tsp (2 ml)
Onion, sliced	1 cup (250 ml)
Parsley	2 tbsp (30 ml)
Garlic clove, minced	1
Water	1 ½ cup (375 ml)
Broccoli, cauliflower or green beans	3 cups (750 ml)
Salt	1 tbsp (15 ml)
Black pepper	½ tsp (2 ml)

For one serving:

Carbohydrates:	11 g = 3 units
Fat:	7 g = 1.5 units
Proteins:	50 g
Calories:	306

Almond Chicken

In bowl, combine half of the cornstarch and soy sauce; mix well. Add chicken and toss to coat. Set aside. Stir the remaining cornstarch into chicken stock. In heavy skillet, cook the chicken until it is opaque. Remove chicken and add celery, beans, carrots, onions and garlic to skillet. Add water, chicken stock mixture and chicken to pan and cook, stirring, for 3 minutes or until mixture boils and vegetables are tender-crisp. Season with salt and pepper to taste. Sprinkle with toasted almonds. Makes 2 servings.

Chicken, cut into strips	8 oz (240 g)
Cornstarch	2 tsp (10 ml)
Soy sauce, sugar free	1 tbsp (15 ml)
Chicken broth	¼ cup (60 ml)
Fresh celery, thinly sliced	1 cup (250 ml)
Green beans, cut	1 cup (250 ml)
Carrots, thinly sliced	½ cup (125 ml)
Onion, sliced	¼ cup (60 ml)
Garlic clove, minced	1
Water	1 tbsp (15 ml)
Almonds, sliced	1 tbsp (15 ml)
Salt, to taste	
Black pepper, to taste	

For one serving:	
Carbohydrates:	20 g = 5 units
Fat:	4 g = 1 unit
Proteins:	30 g
Calories:	235

❖

Chicken with Fine Herbs

Cut chicken in thin strip and put in a non-stick pan with mushrooms. Cook slightly until browned. Add bay leaf, thyme, chervil, parsley, pepper, chicken consommé and water. Cook on medium heat for 10 minutes. Serve very hot. Makes 1 serving.

Chicken	4 oz (120 g)
Fresh mushrooms, minced	5
Bay leaf	1
Thyme	
Chervil	
Consommé, fat free (chicken)	1 tsp (5 ml)
Water	½ cup (125 ml)
Black pepper	

For one serving:

Carbohydrates:	4 g = 1 unit
Fat:	3 g = 0.5 unit
Proteins:	27 g
Calories:	150

❖

Mandarin Chicken

In a non-stick pan, brown chicken on both sides. Remove from pan and set aside. In the same pan, cook mushrooms on high heat. Stirring often. Add water, orange concentrate and instant broth. Bring to a boil, stirring often. Reduce heat, add chicken and let simmer for 3 minutes to blend flavors. Before serving, sprinkle with onions and garnish with mandarins. Makes 2 servings.

Chicken, boneless	4 oz (120 g)
Fresh mushrooms, sliced	1 cup (250 ml)
Flour	1 tsp (5 ml)
Water	¼ cup (60 ml)
Orange juice	⅓ cup (80 ml)
Chicken broth, fat free	½ tsp (2 ml)
Onion, thinly sliced	¼ cup (60 ml)
Mandarin	½ cup (125 ml)

For one serving:

Carbohydrates:	18 g = 4.5 units
Fat:	2 g = 0.5 unit
Proteins:	15 g
Calories:	140

❖

Chicken with Peaches

In a casserole, stir together soy sauce, water, onion, ginger and garlic. Marinate 2 or 3 hours. Mix seasonings and sprinkle over chicken. Bake at a 350 °F/180 °C for 50 minutes, basting several times. Add peaches and water chestnuts. Bake until chicken is tender. Serve with rice. Makes 4 servings.

Soy sauce, sugar free	¼ cup (60 ml)
Water	¼ cup (60 ml)
Onion, chopped	½ cup (125 ml)
Ginger	1 ½ tsp (7 ml)
Garlic clove, finely chopped	1
Chicken, cut up	1 lb (454 g)
Poultry seasoning, ground allspice	¼ tsp (1 ml)
Cinnamon	½ tsp (2 ml)
Peaches quartered	2
Clove	1 pinch
Water chestnut	16 oz (480 g)

For one serving:

Carbohydrates:	10 g = 2.5 units
Fat:	3 g = 0.5 unit
Proteins:	25 g
Calories:	170

❖

Chicken with Fresh Peach

In a baking dish, stir together soy sauce, water, onion, ginger and garlic; add chicken in a single layer; marinate 2 or 3 hours, turning several times. Turn chicken skin side up. Stir together anise, cinnamon and cloves; sprinkle over chicken. Bake in a pre-heated 350 °F/180 °C oven for 40 minutes, basting several times; add peach. Bake until chicken is tender and peach is heated through (10 minutes). Makes 2 servings.

Soy sauce, sugar free	2 tbsp (30 ml)
Water	2 tbsp (30 ml)
Onion, finely chopped	¼ cup (60 ml)
Ginger (fresh), chopped	1 tsp (5 ml)
Garlic clove, chopped	1
Chicken, sliced	8 oz (240 g)
Anise seed, crushed	1 pinch
Cinnamon	¼ tsp (1 ml)
Clove	1 pinch
Peaches (fresh), quartered	1 large

For one serving:
Carbohydrates: 21 g = 5 units
Fat: 4 g = 1 unit
Proteins: 25 g
Calories: 170

❖

Chicken with Apple

Peel off skin and remove fat from chicken breasts. Put them in a baking dish. Add broth, apple slices and celery. Sprinkle with cinnamon and cover. Bake at 425 °F/220 °C for 45 minutes. Sprinkle with chicken broth occasionally. Garnish with parsley before serving. Makes 2 servings.

Chicken breasts	2 of 4 oz (120 g)
Chicken broth	¼ cup (60 ml)
Apples, sliced	2
Fresh celery, chopped	½ cup (125 ml)
Cinnamon	½ tsp (2 ml)

For one serving:

Carbohydrates:	12 g = 3 units
Fat:	8 g = 1.5 units
Proteins:	24 g
Calories:	174

❖

Yogurt and Mushroom Chicken

Remove skin from chicken. Sprinkle chicken lightly with flour. In non-stick skillet, melt butter over medium-high heat; cook chicken until browned all over, about 5 minutes on each side. Reduce heat to medium or medium-low and cook for 10 minutes longer on each side or until meat is no longer pink. Add onions and mushrooms to pan and cook, stirring often, until tender. Stir in water and bring to a boil, loosening any brown bits on bottom of pan to flavor sauce. Remove from heat and stir in yogurt, season to taste. Return chicken and spoon sauce over it. Makes 2 servings.

Chicken breasts	2 of 4 oz (120 g)
Flour	1 tsp (5 ml)
Butter	1 tsp (5 ml)
Onion, thinly sliced	1 small
Fresh mushrooms, sliced	1 cup (250 ml)
Water	¼ cup (60 ml)
Plain yogurt, 2 %	¼ cup (60 ml)
Salt, to taste	
Black pepper, to taste	

For one serving:

Carbohydrates:	10 g = 2.5 units
Fat:	5 g = 1 unit
Proteins:	29 g
Calories:	201

❖

Chicken Basquaise

In a non-stick pan, slightly cook the chicken until browned, with onion and green pepper. Put the chicken, onion and green pepper in a casserole. Add tomato, tomato paste and water. Add a little salt and pepper. Cover and let simmer on low heat for 30 minutes. Sprinkle with parsley before serving. Makes 1 serving.

Chicken	4 oz (120 g)
Onion, finely chopped	1
Green pepper, thin strips	½
Tomato, cut	1 medium
Tomato paste	1 tbsp (15 ml)
Water	2 tbsp (30 ml)
Parsley, chopped, to taste	
Salt, to taste	
Black pepper, to taste	

For one serving:

Carbohydrates:	28 g = 7 units
Fat:	4 g = 1 unit
Proteins:	27 g
Calories:	244

❖

Chicken Brunswick

In a non-stick pan, brown onion until tender. Add chicken. Sprinkle with Worcestershire sauce, cayenne pepper and mustard. Add tomatoes, water. Mix well and bring to a boil. Reduce heat, cover and let simmer for 30 minutes. Add cubed potatoes, green beans, salt and pepper. Simmer, uncovered, for 10 to 15 minutes or until chicken is tender. Makes 2 servings.

Chicken, boneless	8 oz (240 g)
Onion, chopped	¼ cup (60 ml)
Worcestershire sauce	1 tsp (5 ml)
Mustard, dry or Dijon	¼ tsp (1 ml)
Cayenne pepper	¼ tsp (1 ml)
Tomatoes (canned)	½ cup (125 ml)
Water, hot	½ cup (125 ml)
Potato, cubed and cooked	½ cup (125 ml)
Green beans, cut	½ cup (125 ml)
Salt, to taste	
Black pepper, to taste	

For one serving:

Carbohydrates:	22 g = 4.5 units
Fat:	3 g = 0.5 unit
Proteins:	26 g
Calories:	219

❖

Wild Chicken

Place all ingredients except salt, in microwave-safe dish. Micro-wave, covered, at medium-high for 6 ½ minutes. Let stand 4 minutes. Add little salt and serve. Makes 1 serving.

Chicken	4 oz (120 g)
Water	¼ cup (60 ml)
White wine	1 tsp (5 ml)
Fresh mushrooms, minced	4
Onion, chopped	1 tbsp (15 ml)
Consommé (onion)	½ tsp (2 ml)
Tomato paste	1 tsp (5 ml)
Fine herbs, to taste	
Salt, to taste	
Black pepper, to taste	

For one serving:
Carbohydrates: 6 g = 1.5 units
Fat: 2 g = 0.5 unit
Proteins: 27 g
Calories: 161

❖

Stuffed Chicken

Place chicken breast between wax paper sheet and pound with a knife. Spread mustard on the chicken and sprinkle with fine herbs. Stuff chicken with cubed zucchini. Make a roll and secure it with toothpicks. Put in a microwave-safe dish. Sprinkle with pepper. Add chicken consommé and cover. Microwave at medium-high for 4 minutes (70 %). Let stand 3 minutes and serve. Makes 1 serving.

Chicken	4 oz (120 g)
Zucchini, cubed	⅓ cup (80 ml)
Fine herbs	¼ tsp (1 ml)
Dijon mustard	½ tsp (2 ml)
Consommé, fat free (chicken)	2 tbsp (30 ml)
Black pepper, to taste	

For one serving:

Carbohydrates:	2 g = 0.5 unit
Fat:	2 g = 0.5 unit
Proteins:	26 g
Calories:	135

❖

Chicken Gumbo

Simmer all ingredients together until okra is tender. Makes 1 serving.

Chicken, cooked	4 oz (120 g)
Tomatoes, peeled and chopped	1 large
Okra, chopped	½ cup (125 ml)
Shallot, chopped	2
Chicken broth	1 cup (250 ml)

For one serving:

Carbohydrates:	8 g = 2 units
Fat:	14 g = 3 units
Proteins:	26 g
Calories:	265

Chicken Jardinière

In a casserole, place carrot slices, green beans and cubed turnip. Add boiling water (to cover) and cook for 8 to 10 minutes or until vegetables are crisp and tender. Brown onion and chicken. Drain vegetables and keep ½ cup/125 ml from vegetable pan juice. Add vegetables, pan juice and chicken consommé to chicken. Sprinkle with rosemary and pepper. Simmer on low heat for 10 minutes. Sprinkle with parsley before serving. Makes 1 serving.

Chicken, cubed	4 oz (120 g)
Onion, finely chopped	2 tbsp (30 ml)
Carrots, sliced	½ cup (125 ml)
Green beans	½ cup (125 ml)
Turnip, cut into cubes	½ cup (125 ml)
Consommé (chicken)	2 tsp (10 ml)
Rosemary, to taste	
Parsley, chopped, to taste	
Black pepper, to taste	

For one serving:
Carbohydrates: 21 g = 5 units
Fat: 3 g = 0.5 unit
Proteins: 26 g
Calories: 216

❖

Chicken and Vegetables

Debone chicken and put in a microwave-safe dish. Add all vegetables and remaining ingredients. Microwave at full power (high) for 18 minutes. Makes 2 servings.

Chicken breasts	2 of 4 oz (120 g)
Onion, sliced	½ cup (125 ml)
Zucchini	¼ cup (60 ml)
Carrots, sliced	¼ cup (60 ml)
Cauliflower	¼ cup (60 ml)
Fresh celery, chopped	¼ cup (60 ml)
Green beans	½ cup (125 ml)
Fresh mushrooms, sliced	½ cup (125 ml)
Worcestershire sauce	½ tsp (2 ml)
Savory	½ tsp (2 ml)
Thyme	½ tsp (2 ml)
Parsley, chopped	1 tsp (5 ml)
Water	1 ½ cup (375 ml)
Garlic clove	2
Black pepper, to taste	

For one serving:
Carbohydrates: 11 g = 3 units
Fat: 2 g = 0.5 unit
Proteins: 28 g
Calories: 178

❖

Chicken Maria

Place chicken in microwave-safe dish. Add Worcestershire sauce, water, consommé and ginger. Microwave at medium-high (70 %) for 2 minutes. Add shallot and cubed peach and microwave again at medium-high for 2 minutes. Let stand 5 minutes and serve. Makes 1 serving.

Peaches (canned), rinsed	2 pieces
Shallot, chopped	1
Chicken	4 oz (120 g)
Worcestershire sauce	1 tsp (5 ml)
Water	¼ cup (60 ml)
Consommé (chicken)	¼ tsp (1 ml)
Ginger	1 pinch

For one serving:

Carbohydrates:	20 g = 5 units
Fat:	14 g = 3 units
Proteins:	26 g
Calories:	310

❖

Chicken Rice with Fruit

In a casserole, combine rice, broth and raisins. Bring to a boil and place mixture in baking dish. Season. Add chicken to the rice dish and cover. Bake at 325 °F/160 °C for 45 minutes. Add apples and bake uncovered for 10 minutes. Makes 2 servings.

Rice (brown), cooked	¼ cup (60 ml)
Chicken broth, fat free	½ cup (125 ml)
Raisins	2 tbsp (30 ml)
Nutmeg	1 pinch
Chicken breasts	2 of 4 oz (120 g)
Apple (peeled), cubed	1
Cinnamon	½ tsp (2 ml)
Salt, to taste	
Black pepper, to taste	

For one serving:

Carbohydrates:	35 g = 9 units	
Fat:	3 g = 0.5 unit	
Proteins:	28 g	
Calories:	279	

❖

Turkey Roast with Fine Herbs

Mix all ingredients and pour over turkey. Bake at 350 °F/180 °C
for 2 hours, baste often during baking. Makes 6 servings.

Turkey roast	4 lbs (1.8 kg)
Salt	½ tsp (2 ml)
Sage	¼ tsp (1 ml)
Water	¼ cup (60 ml)
Vinegar	¾ cup (180 ml)
Thyme	¼ tsp (1 ml)
Black pepper	¼ tsp (1 ml)

For one serving:
Carbohydrates: 20 g = 4 units
Fat: 7 g = 1.5 units
Proteins: 53 g
Calories: 360

❖

Chicken Steak

Pound the chicken to tenderize it. Pour half of the Worcestershire sauce on the breasts and add seasoning. Tenderize until
the chicken is thin and flat. Broil both sides and add the rest of
the sauce. Makes 1 serving.

Chicken, boneless	4 oz (120 g)
Worcestershire sauce	1 tsp (5 ml)
Garlic clove, minced	1
Italian seasoning	¼ tsp (1 ml)
Poultry seasoning	¼ tsp (1 ml)
Salt	1 pinch
Black pepper, to taste	

For one serving:
Carbohydrates: 1 g
Fat: 2 g = 0.5 unit
Proteins: 26 g
Calories: 131

Haddock with Celery

Microwave, celery and onion covered at full power for 2 minutes. Add fillet, salt and pepper. Sprinkle with lemon juice and microwave, covered, at full power for 1 ½ minute. Let stand 2 to 3 minutes. Sprinkle with fresh chopped parsley. Makes 1 serving.

Haddock fillet	4 oz (120 g)
Fresh celery, cubed	½ cup (125 ml)
Onion, minced	1 tbsp (15 ml)
Lemon juice	2 tbsp (30 ml)
Parsley, chopped, to taste	
Salt and black pepper, to taste	

For one serving:
Carbohydrates: 8 g = 2 units
Fat: 1 g
Proteins: 23 g
Calories: 129

❖

Haddock Bonne-Femme

Put fillet of haddock in a microwave-safe dish. Add vegetables and sprinkle with lemon juice. Cover and microwave at full power for 2 minutes. Let stand 3 minutes and place fillet in serving dish. Mix yogurt with pan juices and pour on fish. Sprinkle with peppercorns and serve with lemon wedges. Makes 1 serving.

Haddock fillet	4 oz (120 g)
Lemon juice	1 tsp (5 ml)
Fresh mushrooms, minced	2
Onion, chopped	1 tbsp (15 ml)
Plain yogurt, 2 %	1 tbsp (15 ml)
Peppercorns, to taste	
Lemon, sliced, to taste	

For one serving:	
Carbohydrates:	9 g = 2 units
Fat:	Trace amount
Proteins:	24 g
Calories:	141

❖

Bouillabaisse Gaspésienne

In a non-stick pan, brown onion, celery and garlic before placing in a casserole. Add tomatoes, fish and fine herbs, saffron and water. Cook on medium heat for 10 minutes. Then, add lobster and onion in powder. Simmer on low heat for 10 minutes. Serve hot. Makes 2 servings.

Boston bluefish	4 oz (120 g)
Tomatoes (canned)	½ cup (125 ml)
Onion, finely chopped	1 small
Fresh celery, diced	½ cup (125 ml)
Garlic clove, chopped	1
Lobster (canned)	4 oz (120 g)
Oregano	1 tsp (5 ml)
Water	1 cup (250 ml)
Saffron (in powder)	½ tsp (2 ml)
Onion (in powder)	1 tsp (5 ml)

For one serving:
Carbohydrates: 12 g = 3 units
Fat: 1 g
Proteins: 22 g
Calories: 149

❖

Seafood Brochette (1)

Make the marinade with lemon juice and seasonings. Let shrimp and scallops marinate for at least 2 hours. Remove scallops and shrimp and keep marinade. On skewer, thread shrimp and scallops alternating with tomato and green pepper. Bake 15 minutes, brushing the brochette with marinade while cooking. Makes 1 serving.

Scallops	2 oz (60 g)
Shrimp	1 oz (30 g)
Tomato wedges	1
Green pepper, cut	½ cup (125 ml)
Lemon juice	2 tsp (10 ml)
Water	2 tbsp (30 ml)
Black pepper and salt, to taste	

For one serving:

Carbohydrates:	16 g = 4 units
Fat:	2 g = 0.5 unit
Proteins:	16 g
Calories:	141

❖

Seafood Brochette (2)

Marinate shrimp and scallops in the lemon juice and seasonings. Drain and keep the sauce. On a skewer, alternate the scallops, shrimp, green pepper and tomato. Place the brochette on the grill. Cook 15 minutes. Turn and brush the brochette with the remaining sauce. Makes 1 serving.

Scallops fresh or frozen	1 ½ oz (45 g)
Shrimp fresh	1 oz (30 g)
Lemon juice	2 tsp (10 ml)
Water	2 tsp (10 ml)
Tomatoes quarters	½ cup (125 ml)
Green pepper pieces	½ cup (125 ml)
Black pepper, to taste	

For one serving:

Carbohydrates:	15 g = 4 units	
Fat:	2 g = 0.5 unit	
Proteins:	19 g	
Calories:	147	

❖

Baked Salmon with Curry

Drain salmon (keep juice) and cut into large cubes. In a non-stick pan, brown all vegetables and add a part of the salmon juice and skimmed milk. Cook for a few minutes then sprinkle with curry and pepper. Add salmon and mix. Pour the mixture into a baking dish and sprinkle with grated cheese. Bake at 400 °F/205 °C for 10 minutes or until cheese melts. Makes 1 serving.

Salmon, canned	4 oz (120 g)
Onion finely, chopped	1
Fresh celery, cubed	¼ cup (60 ml)
Green pepper, cubed	¼ cup (60 ml)
Skimmed milk	¼ cup (60 ml)
Curry	1 tsp (5 ml)
Cheese, grated	2 tbsp (30 ml)
Black pepper, to taste	

For one serving:

Carbohydrates:	20 g	= 5 units
Fat:	22 g	= 4.5 units
Proteins:	37 g	
Calories:	396	

❖

Fish Casserole with Tomato

In a non-stick pan, combine all ingredients except fish. Let simmer on low heat for about 20 minutes or until green pepper is tender. Add fish fillet and simmer until fish flakes. Makes 1 serving.

Tomato, peeled and sliced	1
Sole fillet	4 oz (120 g)
Green pepper, chopped	¼ cup (60 ml)
Thyme	¼ tsp (1 ml)
Onion, chopped	1 tbsp (15 ml)
Salt	¼ tsp (1 ml)
Black pepper and Tabasco sauce, to taste	

For one serving:

Carbohydrates:	10 g = 2.5 units
Fat:	2 g = 0.5 unit
Proteins:	23 g
Calories:	148

❖

Fisherman's Chowder

Combine vegetables with seasonings and add boiling water. Bring to a boil. Lower heat and simmer 10 minutes. Add salmon and shrimp and simmer 5 minutes more. In a skillet, melt butter, add flour and mix well. Gradually add milk and cook a few minutes while stirring until sauce thickens. Add vegetables and fish to sauce, stir and garnish with parsley. Makes 2 servings.

Potato, cubed	½ cup (125 ml)
Water, boiling	½ cup (125 ml)
Onion, sliced	¼ cup (60 ml)
Tomatoes, cubed	⅓ cup (80 ml)
Salmon, cooked and flaked	4 oz (120 g)
Shrimp, cooked	2 oz (60 g)
Butter	1 tsp (5 ml)
Flour, all-purpose	1 tsp (5 ml)
Skim milk	¾ cup (180 ml)
Celery seeds	¼ tsp (1 ml)
Thyme	1 pinch
Parsley, chopped	1 tsp (5 ml)
Black pepper, to taste	

For one serving:

Carbohydrates:	24 g	= 6 units
Fat:	7 g	= 1.5 units
Proteins:	26 g	
Calories:	264	

❖

Coquille St-Jacques, traditional oven

Stir yogurt with scallops and add a little salt, pepper and a dash of basil. Put in a baking dish. Sprinkle with grated cheese and bake at 400 °F/205 °C for 20 minutes or until heated through. Makes 1 serving.

Scallops, chopped	4 oz (120 g)
Plain yogurt, 2 %	2 tbsp (30 ml)
Cheese, grated	2 tbsp (30 ml)
Salt, black pepper and basil, to taste	

For one serving:	
Carbohydrates:	6 g = 1.5 units
Fat:	7 g = 1.5 units
Proteins:	29 g
Calories:	209

❖

Coquille Saint-Jacques, microwave

Place minced mushrooms and shallots in microwave-safe dish. Microwave at full power for 2 minutes. Add scallops, water, thyme and bay leaf. Microwave at full power for 1 ½ minute. Remove bay leaf and pour off pan juices from casserole. Combine yogurt with pan juices and pour over scallops. Sprinkle with grated cheese and microwave at full power for 30 seconds. Serve hot. Makes 1 serving.

Scallops	3 oz (90 g)
Plain yogurt, 2 %	1 tbsp (15 ml)
Shallot, chopped	2 tbsp (30 ml)
Water	2 tbsp (30 ml)
Mozzarella skimmed cheese, grated	1 tbsp (15 ml)
Thyme	¼ tsp (1 ml)
Bay leaf	1
Mushrooms, fresh, minced	3

For one serving:

Carbohydrates:	6 g = 1.5 units
Fat:	4 g = 1 unit
Proteins:	22 g
Calories:	150

❖

Salmon Steak with Dill

Place salmon steak in microwave-safe dish. Add onion, lemon juice, consommé, water and dill. Microwave, covered, at full power for 3 minutes.

SAUCE:

Combine all the remaining ingredients and microwave at full power for 30 seconds. Top salmon steak with sauce and serve. Makes 1 serving.

Salmon steak	4 oz (120 g)
Onion slices	3
Consommé (chicken)	½ tsp (2 ml)
Dill	½ tsp (2 ml)
Water	2 tbsp (30 ml)
Lemon juice	1 tbsp (15 ml)
SAUCE:	
Lemon juice	½ tsp (2 ml)
Plain yogurt, 2 %	1 tbsp (15 ml)
Pan juices	
Dill fresh, to taste	
Salt to taste	
Black pepper, to taste	

For one serving:
Carbohydrates: 2 g = 0.5 unit
Fat: 12 g = 2.5 units
Proteins: 23 g
Calories: 216

❖

Rolled Boston Bluefish

Cut the fish fillet in two, lengthwise. Combine all ingredients to prepare stuffing, then place it on each fish fillet. Roll up fillets and secure with toothpicks. Place the rolls in a baking dish. Bake at 450 °F/230 °C for 15 minutes or until the fish flakes. Makes 1 serving.

Boston bluefish fillet	4 oz (120 g)
Salt and black pepper to taste	
Spinach	2 leaves
STUFFING:	
Lemon juice	1 tsp (5 ml)
Shallot, chopped	1 tbsp (15 ml)
Tomatoes, chopped	¼ cup (60 ml)
Fresh mushrooms, sliced	¼ cup (60 ml)

For one serving:

Carbohydrates:	6 g = 1.5 units
Fat:	Trace amount
Proteins:	23 g
Calories:	131

❖

Halibut with Vegetables

Place the halibut in a baking dish, add salt and pepper. In a bowl combine all other ingredients and mix well. Top halibut with this mixture. Cover with a piece of foil and bake at 450 °F/230 °C for 15 minutes. Remove foil and bake for 10 more minutes. Serve. Makes 1 serving.

Halibut	4 oz (120 g)
Fresh mushrooms, minced	½ cup (125 ml)
Shallot, chopped	2
Tomato paste	1 tsp (5 ml)
Worcestershire sauce	1 tsp (5 ml)
Water	1 tbsp (15 ml)
Salt and black pepper, to taste	

For one serving:
Carbohydrates: 6 g = 1.5 units
Fat: 3 g = 0.5 unit
Proteins: 26 g
Calories: 155

❖

Halibut with Lemon

Place the fish fillet in a baking dish. Top with crushed coriander seeds, green and red pepper, lemon juice, salt and pepper. Cover with foil. Bake at 350 °F/180 °C for 10 minutes or until the fish flakes. Makes 1 serving.

Halibut fillet	4 oz (120 g)
Coriander seeds, crushed	6
Red pepper, chopped	¼ cup (60 ml)
Green pepper, chopped	¼ cup (60 ml)
Lemon juice	2 tbsp (30 ml)
Water	2 tbsp (30 ml)
Salt and black pepper, to taste	

For one serving:
Carbohydrates: 7 g = 2 units
Fat: 3 g = 0.5 unit
Proteins: 24 g
Calories: 151

❖

Portuguese Cod Fillet

In a non-stick pan, cook onion and garlic until tender. Add the green pepper and cook 3 minutes more then add tomatoes, wine and olives. Cover and let simmer for 10 minutes. Stir occasionally. In a non-stick pan, cook the fish for 3 to 4 minutes and add salt and pepper. Turn the fillet, top with vegetables and simmer for 3 minutes or until fish flakes. Place fish in serving dish. Makes 2 servings.

Cod fillet	8 oz (240 g)
Onion, chopped	¼ cup (60 ml)
Garlic clove, chopped	1
Green pepper, cubed	½ cup (125 ml)
Tomatoes (canned)	¾ cup (180 ml)
White wine (dry)	2 tbsp (30 ml)
Olive (black), sliced	4
Parsley (fresh), chopped	2 tsp (10 ml)
Salt and black pepper, to taste	

For one serving:

Carbohydrates:	13 g = 3 units
Fat:	4 g = 1 unit
Proteins:	21 g
Calories:	160

❖

Cod with Vegetables

Place tomato cut into wedges, green pepper, onion, mushrooms and grated lemon in microwave dish. Microwave, covered, at full power for 2 minutes. Add cod, thyme, lemon juice, salt and pepper. Microwave, covered, at full power for 2 ½ minutes. Sprinkle with parsley. Makes 1 serving.

Cod fillet	4 oz (120 g)
Lemon zest	1 tsp (5 ml)
Lemon juice	1 tbsp (15 ml)
Tomato (canned)	1
Green pepper, minced	2 tbsp (30 ml)
Onion, minced	1 tbsp (15 ml)
Fresh mushrooms, minced	1 cup (250 ml)
Thyme	¼ tsp (1 ml)
Salt, black pepper and parsley, to taste	

For one serving:

Carbohydrates:	18 g = 4.5 units
Fat:	1 g
Proteins:	23 g
Calories:	169

❖

Cod Bergeronne

Place tomato cut into wedges in microwave-safe dish. Cut fillet of cod in three pieces and place with tomato. Add lemon slices between each piece of cod. Add garlic, onion and sweet pepper. Sprinkle with parsley and microwave at full power for 2 ½ minutes. Let stand 3 minutes and serve. Makes 1 serving.

Cod fillet	4 oz (120 g)
Onion, sliced	1
Green pepper, cubed	2 tbsp (30 ml)
Lemon, sliced	2
Parsley, chopped	1 tsp (5 ml)
Tomato (canned)	1
Garlic, minced	1 clove
Salt, to taste	

For one serving:
Carbohydrates: 9 g = 2 units
Fat: 1 g
Proteins: 22 g
Calories: 134

❖

Poached Cod and Mushroom Sauce

Place fillet in a baking dish. Add mushrooms and herbs. Mix soup with water and add to fish. Cover and microwave at full power for 3 minutes. Sprinkle with parsley and serve. Makes 1 serving.

Cod fillet	4 oz (120 g)
Water	½ cup (125 ml)
Mushroom cream	1 tsp (5 ml)
Rosemary	¼ tsp (1 ml)
Bay leaf	1
Fresh mushrooms	1 cup (250 ml)
Parsley, to taste	

For one serving:

Carbohydrates:	15 g = 4 units
Fat:	5 g = 1 unit
Proteins:	25 g
Calories:	197

❖

Pescado à la Naranja (halibut)

Arrange fish in baking dish. In small non-stick pan, cook onion and garlic until onion is tender. Stir in spices. Spread mixture over fish. Combine orange juice with lemon juice and pour over fish. Cover and bake at 400 °F/205 °C for 15 to 20 minutes. Arrange egg slices on top of fish and sprinkle with paprika. Makes 1 serving.

Halibut	4 oz (120 g)
Onion, chopped	1 tbsp (15 ml)
Garlic clove, chopped	1
Parsley, chopped	½ tsp (2 ml)
Orange juice	1 tbsp (15 ml)
Egg, hard boiled	3 slices
Lemon juice	½ tsp (2 ml)
Paprika	
Salt and black pepper, to taste	

For one serving:
Carbohydrates: 5 g = 1 unit
Fat: 8 g = 1.5 units
Proteins: 30 g
Calories: 215

❖

Baked Salmon

Place salmon steak in a baking dish. Sprinkle with lemon juice, top with shallots and seasonings. Bake at 375 °F/190 °C for 25 to 35 minutes or until the fish flakes. Serve with lemon slices and garnish with parsley. Makes 1 serving.

Salmon steak	4 oz (120 g)
Lemon juice	1 tbsp (15 ml)
Shallot, chopped	2 tbsp (30 ml)
Lemon	1 slice
Parsley, chopped	1 pinch

For one serving:
Carbohydrates: 4 g = 1 unit
Fat: 12 g = 2.5 units
Proteins: 23 g
Calories: 219

❖

Salmon with Shrimp

In a microwave dish, place salmon with shrimp. Add water, wine, shallot and fine herbs. Microwave at full power for 3 minutes. Remove salmon and shrimp from baking dish. Add a little salt and pepper to pan juices. Add cornstarch mixed with cold water. Microwave at full power for 30 seconds and top salmon with mixture. Makes 1 serving.

Salmon steak	3 oz (90 g)
Shrimp	1 oz (30 g)
Lemon juice	1 tbsp (15 ml)
White wine	1 tsp (5 ml)
Shallot, chopped	1
Thyme	¼ tsp (1 ml)
Parsley, chopped	½ tsp (2 ml)
Cornstarch	¼ tsp (1 ml)
Water (cold)	1 tbsp (15 ml)
Salt, to taste	
Black pepper, to taste	

For one serving:	
Carbohydrates:	3 g = 1 unit
Fat:	10 g = 2 units
Proteins:	23 g
Calories:	196

❖

Fish Fillet à la Créole (1)

Heat oven to 450 °F/230 °C. Cut fish fillet into 2 servings and season. Bake for 25 to 35 minutes. Cook celery and shallot in a non-stick pan. Add tomatoes, oregano, basil and let simmer for 5 minutes. Mix cornstarch and cold water and add to the sauce. Cook until it thickens. Pour tomato sauce on the cooked fish. Sprinkle with bread crumbs and broil until browned. Makes 2 servings.

Sole fillet	8 oz (240 g)
Fresh celery, cubed	¼ cup (60 ml)
Shallot, chopped	1
Tomatoes (canned)	½ cup (125 ml)
Oregano	½ tsp (2 ml)
Basil	½ tsp (2 ml)
Cornstarch	2 tsp (10 ml)
Water (cold)	1 tbsp (15 ml)
Bread crumbs	⅓ cup (80 ml)
Salt and black pepper, to taste	

For one serving:

Carbohydrates:	25 g = 6 units
Fat:	2 g = 0.5 unit
Proteins:	26 g
Calories:	237

❖

Fish Créole (2)

Arrange the fillets in a lightly greased square pan. In a frying pan cook onion and celery in butter until tender. Stir in remaining ingredients and mix well. Pour tomato mixture over fillets and bake uncovered at 350 °F/180 °C for 30-35 minutes. Makes 3 servings.

Sole or other fish	1 lb (454 g)
Butter	1 tsp (5 ml)
Onion	1
Fresh celery, diced	½ cup (125 ml)
Tomatoes	1 cup (250 ml)
Green pepper, chopped	2 tbsp (30 ml)
Oregano	¼ tsp (1 ml)
Sugar substitute, to taste	
Salt	½ tsp (2 ml)
Black pepper	1 pinch

For one serving:

Carbohydrates:	8 g = 2 units
Fat:	4 g = 1 unit
Proteins:	30 g
Calories:	187

❖

Fish Fillet with Orange

Place fish fillet in a non-stick pan. Add grated orange rind, orange juice and sprinkle with nutmeg. Cover with a piece of foil and bake at 450 °F/230 °C for 10 to 15 minutes. Serve and garnish with parsley. Makes 1 serving.

Sole fillet	4 oz (120 g)
Orange juice	¼ cup (60 ml)
Orange zest	1 tbsp (15 ml)
Nutmeg	1 tsp (5 ml)
Parsley	
Mint, chopped	2 tsp (10 ml)

For one serving:
Carbohydrates: 8 g = 2 units
Fat: 1 g
Proteins: 22 g
Calories: 138

❖

Fish Fillet Provençal

In a non-stick pan, place the fish fillet. Add sliced mushrooms and a dash of basil and chervil. Mix the tomato juice with onion consommé and add to the fish. Cover with a piece of foil and bake at 450 °F/230 °C for 15 minutes. Makes 1 serving.

Sole fillet	4 oz (120 g)
Fresh mushrooms, sliced	4
Tomato juice	2 tbsp (30 ml)
Consommé (onion), fat free	2 tsp (10 ml)
Chervil, basil and black pepper, to taste	

For one serving:
Carbohydrates: 5 g = 1 unit
Fat: 2 g = 0.5 unit
Proteins: 23 g
Calories: 125

Alsatian Sole

In a baking dish, spread the sauerkraut and place the sole fillet on top. Sprinkle with cumin and pepper. Cover with a piece of foil and bake at 400 °F/205 °C for 8 to 10 minutes. Sprinkle with parsley and serve. Makes 1 serving.

Sauerkraut, canned	½ cup (125 ml)
Sole fillet	4 oz (120 g)
Cumin, to taste	
Parsley, chopped, to taste	
Black pepper, to taste	

For one serving:

Carbohydrates:	5 g = 1 unit
Fat:	1 g
Proteins:	13 g
Calories:	126

❖

Baked Sole

Combine all ingredients except sole and shrimp in saucepan. Cook over medium heat until boiling. Boil 1 minute, stir constantly. Place fish in Pam-sprayed baking dish and pour mixture over top. Place shrimp evenly over fillets, cover tightly and bake in pre-heated oven for 20 minutes at 375 °F/190 °C. Makes 4 servings.

Sole fillets	1 lb (454 g)
Lemon juice	2 tbsp (30 ml)
Shrimp	1 cup (250 ml)
Onion, minced	2 tsp (10 ml)
Fresh mushrooms, chopped	1 cup (250 ml)
Water	½ cup (125 ml)
Parsley	1 tbsp (15 ml)
Salt	1 tsp (5 ml)

For one serving:

Carbohydrates:	3 g = 0.5 unit
Fat:	2 g = 0.5 unit
Proteins:	30 g
Calories:	157

❖

Sole with Clams

Place tomatoes, seasonings and Worcestershire sauce in a microwave-safe dish. Microwave covered at medium power (50 %) for 5 minutes. Add clams, sugar substitute and mix well. In another microwave dish, place sole fillet and microwave at full power for 5 minutes. Top fish fillet with hot clam sauce. Makes 2 servings.

Sole fillet	8 oz (240 g)
Tomatoes, peeled (crunched)	¾ cup (180 ml)
Garlic clove	2
Clams (canned)	½ cup (125 ml)
Parsley, chopped	1 tsp (5 ml)
Basil	1 tsp (5 ml)
Worcestershire sauce	½ tsp (2 ml)
Cayenne pepper, to taste	
Sugar substitute	½ tsp (2 ml)
Black pepper, to taste	

For one serving:

Carbohydrates:	6 g = 1.5 units
Fat:	3 g = 0.5 unit
Proteins:	34 g
Calories:	194

❖

Fillet of Sole Dieppoise

Place fillet of sole, shrimp, mushrooms and wine in microwave-safe dish. Microwave at full power for 1 ½ minute. Place fillet of sole in serving dish. Blend yogurt into pan juice and top fillet with this mixture. Sprinkle with parsley and serve. Makes 1 serving.

Sole fillet	3 oz (90 g)
Shrimp (cooked)	1 oz (30 g)
Fresh mushrooms, minced	2
Plain yogurt, 2 %	1 tbsp (15 ml)
White wine	½ tsp (2 ml)
Parsley, chopped	

For one serving:

Carbohydrates:	4 g = 1 unit
Fat:	2 g = 0.5 unit
Proteins:	27 g
Calories:	148

❖

Sole Dijonnaise

Brush fish fillet with mustard and place it in a glass dish. Top fish with green peppers and onion. Then, add milk and lemon juice. Sprinkle with grated cheese and paprika. Bake at 375 °F/190 °C for 15 minutes or until fish flakes. Makes 2 servings.

Sole fillet	8 oz (240 g)
Dijon mustard	1 tbsp (15 ml)
Green pepper, cubed	½ cup (125 ml)
Onion, chopped	¼ cup (60 ml)
Milk, 2 %	2 tbsp (30 ml)
Lemon juice	2 tsp (10 ml)
Low fat cheese, grated	¼ cup (10 ml)
Paprika, to taste	

For one serving:

Carbohydrates:	8 g = 2 units
Fat:	10 g = 2 units
Proteins:	30 g
Calories:	245

❖

Doria Sole

Place sole fillet in microwave-safe dish and add all other ingredients. Cover and microwave at full power for 2 ½ minutes. Let stand 3 minutes.

SAUCE:

Microwave tomato sauce and yogurt at full power for 20 seconds and add tarragon. Place sole fillet in a serving dish and top with sauce. Makes 1 serving.

Sole fillet	4 oz (120 g)
Cucumber, sliced	10 slices
Lemon juice	1 tsp (5 ml)
Worcestershire sauce	1 tsp (5 ml)
Thyme	¼ tsp (1 ml)
Parsley, fresh	¼ tsp (1 ml)
Onion, minced	1 tbsp (15 ml)
SAUCE:	
Tomato paste	1 tsp (5 ml)
Plain yogurt, 2 %	1 tbsp (15 ml)
Tarragon, to taste	

For one serving:
Carbohydrates: 9 g = 2 units
Fat: 2 g = 0.5 unit
Proteins: 24 g
Calories: 149

❖

Sole Fillet en Verdure

Place broccoli in baking dish, stems outside. Add water and microwave at full power for 3 minutes. Place fillet of sole on broccoli and add fine herbs. Cover and microwave at full power for 2 ½ minutes and let stand 4 minutes. Serve with lemon and sprinkle with lemon juice. Makes 1 serving.

Sole fillet	4 oz (120 g)
Broccoli	⅔ cup (160 ml)
Water	2 tbsp (30 ml)
Tarragon	¼ tsp (1 ml)
Parsley	¼ tsp (1 ml)
Shallot, chopped	¼ tsp (1 ml)
Lemon wedges	2

For one serving:

Carbohydrates:	20 g = 5 units
Fat:	2 g = 0.5 unit
Proteins:	30 g
Calories:	204

❖

Sole Fillet Gratiné

Place the fish fillet in a baking dish. Season with onions, garlic, oregano, salt and pepper. Cover with tomato slices. Bake at 375 °F/190 °C for 10 minutes or until the fish flakes. When the fish is cooked, top it with grated cheese. Grill 2 or 3 minutes until cheese has browned. Makes 1 serving.

Sole fillet	4 oz (120 g)
Onion, finely chopped	1 tbsp (15 ml)
Tomato, sliced	1 small
Low fat cheese, grated	3 tbsp (45 ml)
Garlic powder	½ tsp (2 ml)
Oregano	¼ tsp (1 ml)
Salt and black pepper, to taste	

For one serving:
Carbohydrates: 9 g = 2 units
Fat: 10 g = 2 units
Proteins: 35 g
Calories: 272

❖

Sole Fillet Marinière

Place sole fillet in a lightly greased baking dish. Combine in non-stick pan: tomato, capers and parsley. Add salt, pepper and oregano. Cook on medium heat for a few minutes. Stir once. Pour tomato onto fish fillet and cover with a piece of foil. Bake at 450 °F/230 ° for 15 minutes. Serve. Makes 1 serving.

Sole fillet	4 oz (120 g)
Tomato (fresh)	1
Capers	1 tbsp (15 ml)
Parsley, chopped	1 tbsp (15 ml)
Oregano	¼ tsp (1 ml)
Salt and black pepper, to taste	

For one serving:
Carbohydrates: 6 g = 1.5 units
Fat: 2 g = 1 unit
Proteins: 22 g
Calories: 128

❖

Sole Niçoise

Place sole fillet in a baking dish. In another bowl, combine crushed tomato, chopped garlic clove, basil and some capers. Pour the mixture over fillet of sole. Cover and microwave at full power for 2 ½ minutes. Let stand 3 minutes before serving. Makes 1 serving.

Sole fillet	4 oz (120 g)
Tomato fresh	1
Basil	¼ tsp (1 ml)
Garlic clove, chopped	1
Capers, to taste	

For one serving:
Carbohydrates: 7 g = 2 units
Fat: 2 g = 0.5 unit
Proteins: 22 g
Calories: 132

Provençal Tuna (1)

Place tuna carefully in a baking dish. Sprinkle it with lemon juice. Add salt and pepper. In a non-stick pan, cook onions until they are tender. Add garlic, tomatoes, water, salt and pepper. Let boil until mixture thickens. Pour tomato mixture on tuna and cover. Bake at 350 °F/180 °C for 10 minutes. Garnish with parsley before serving. Makes 2 servings.

Tuna, drained	6 oz (180 g)
Onion, chopped	½ cup (125 ml)
Garlic clove, crushed	1
Tomatoes, peeled	1 cup (250 ml)
Water	½ cup (125 ml)
Lemon juice	2 tbsp (30 ml)
Parsley and oregano	½ tsp (2 ml) each
Capers, rinsed	½ tsp (2 ml)
Salt and black pepper	1 pinch

For one serving:

Carbohydrates:	10 g = 2.5 units
Fat:	3 g = 2 units
Proteins:	21 g
Calories:	150

❖

Provençal Tuna (2)

In a non-stick pan, brown onions and garlic until the onions are tender. Add eggplant, tomatoes, green peppers, water, basil, oregano and pepper. Cover and simmer for 35 minutes. Stir in tuna and simmer for 5 minutes longer. Before serving, sprinkle with parsley. Makes 2 servings.

Tuna, drained	6 oz (180 g)
Eggplant, cubed	2 cups (500 ml)
Onion sliced	1 cup (250 ml)
Garlic clove, chopped	1
Tomatoes, canned	2 cups (500 ml)
Green pepper, sliced	1 cup (250 ml)
Water	1 cup (250 ml)
Basil	½ tsp (2 ml)
Oregano	¼ tsp (1 ml)
Parsley (fresh), chopped	2 tsp (10 ml)
Black pepper	1 pinch

For one serving:
Carbohydrates: 34 g = 8.5 units
Fat: 4 g = 1 unit
Proteins: 25 g
Calories: 255

Tuna Cucumber Boats

Cut cucumbers in half lengthwise and scoop out seeds. Mix seeds with tomato, onion, and tuna. Spoon mixture into cucumber shells. Pour dressing over top and serve. Makes 2 servings.

Cucumber	1 large
Tomato, diced	1 medium
Onion, diced	¼ cup (60 ml)
Tuna	6 oz (180 g)
Oil	2 tbsp (30 ml)
Balsamic vinegar	1 tbsp (15 ml)
Salt and black pepper, to taste	

For one serving:

Carbohydrates:	6 g	= 1.5 units
Fat:	17 g	= 3.5 units
Proteins:	21 g	
Calories:	259	

❖

Stuffed Eggplant

Cut the eggplants in half, lengthwise. Scoop out some of the flesh and chop fine. Boil the onion in very lightly salted water for 3-4 minutes. Drain well. Add to the eggplant flesh, together with the tomatoes, parsley, mushrooms, oregano, salt and pepper. Mix well and fill each eggplant half with this mixture. Bake at 350 °F/180 °C for 45 minutes. Serve hot or cold. Makes 3 servings.

Eggplant	3
Tomatoes, peeled and chopped	½ cup (125 ml)
Parsley	2 tsp (10 ml)
Oregano	1 tsp (5 ml)
Onion, chopped	1 cup (250 ml)
Fresh mushrooms, chopped	½ cup (125 ml)
Black pepper and salt, to taste	

For one serving:

Carbohydrates:	17 g = 4 units
Fat:	Trace amount
Proteins:	3 g
Calories:	80

❖

Eggplant Marinade

Peel and cut eggplant in cubes. Steam for about 3-5 minutes, making sure eggplant is firm. Marinate overnight in small amount of safflower oil, white vinegar, water, oregano, thyme, basil, garlic powder, onion powder, salt and pepper. Makes 1 serving.

Eggplant	2 cups (500 ml)
Olive oil and white vinegar	1 tsp (5 ml) each
Water, to taste	
Oregano, to taste	
Thyme, to taste	
Basil, to taste	
Garlic powder and onion powder to taste	
Salt and pepper to taste	

For one serving:
Carbohydrates: 26 g = 6.5 units
Fat: 6 g = 1 unit
Proteins: 4 g
Calories: 160

❖

Dilled Zucchini

Cut 2 prepared medium zucchini lengthwise in half. Cook uncovered in 1 inch (2,5 cm) boiling water with salt added, until tender. Drain. Brush with imitation butter flavoring and sprinkle with dill weed. Makes 4 servings.

Zucchini, sliced	2 medium
Water	$\frac{1}{2}$ cup (125 ml)
Dill fresh, to taste	
Salt, to taste	

For one serving:
Carbohydrates: 2 g = 0.5 unit
Fat: 0
Proteins: 1 g
Calories: 10

Squash Bake

Melt butter over low heat, add onion and simmer 2 minutes, then add zucchini and simmer until partly done. Add onion powder, garlic powder and salt. Stir. Add chicken broth. Pour into ovenware and sprinkle with cheese. Bake until cheese is slightly brown. Makes 4 servings.

Zucchini, cubed	4
Chicken broth, fat free	1 tsp (5 ml)
Onion, chopped	½ cup (125 ml)
Cheddar cheese, grated	1 cup (250 ml)
Butter	1 tbsp (15 ml)
Garlic clove, minced	1
Salt	1 tsp (5 ml)
Black pepper	½ tsp (2 ml)

For one serving:

Carbohydrates:	5 g = 1 unit
Fat:	19 g = 4 units
Proteins:	25 g
Calories:	312

❖

Tangy Zucchini

Put onions in oil. Cut zucchini into ¼″ slices. Peel and cut up tomato. Add everything to onion, cook covered for 20 minutes.
Makes 4 servings.

Zucchini, sliced	3 cups (750 ml)
Onion, chopped	¼ cup (60 ml)
Vegetable oil	2 tsp (10 ml)
Chili powder	½ tsp (2 ml)
Tomato peeled	1
Salt	½ tsp (2 ml)
Black pepper	1 pinch

For one serving:

Carbohydrates::	8 g = 2 units
Fat:	3 g = 1 unit
Proteins:	2 g
Calories:	58

Stuffed Zucchini (1)

Carefully peel zucchini and core them with a knife. Combine all the ingredients, stuff the zucchini and shape the remaining mixture into meatballs. In a casserole, mix broth and lemon slices, then add the stuffed squash and the meatballs. Cover and simmer for 30 to 45 minutes. Makes 2 servings.

Zucchini	2
Beef, lean ground	7 oz (210 g)
Onion, chopped	¼ cup (60 ml)
Egg	1
Parsley, chopped (fresh)	2 tbsp (30 ml)
Beef broth	1 cup (250 ml)
Sage	⅛ tsp (0.5 ml)
Lemon	2 slices
Salt and black pepper, to taste	

For one serving:

Carbohydrates:	13 g	= 3 units
Fat:	18 g	= 3.5 units
Proteins:	25 g	
Calories:	320	

❖

Stuffed Zucchini (2)

Halve zucchini lengthwise. Scoop out pulp. Chop pulp to make 1 cup (250 ml); set aside. Place zucchini shells, cut down, in a large skillet. Add water. Simmer, covered, until just tender, 5-6 minutes. Drain. Turn cut side up in the same skillet. Salt. Meanwhile, in a medium skillet cook zucchini pulp and tomato until tender about 3 minutes. Add eggs, pepper and cook at low heat until set. Spoon egg into zucchini shells. Top with cheese. Cover. Heat until cheese melts. Makes 4 servings.

Zucchini, sliced	4 medium
Water	½ cup (125 ml)
Tomato, chopped	1
Eggs, beaten	3
Cheddar cheese, shredded	½ cup (125 ml)
Salt	¼ tsp (1 ml)
Black pepper	1 pinch

For one serving:

Carbohydrates:	6.5 g = 1.5 units
Fat:	15 g = 3 units
Proteins:	15 g
Calories:	214

❖

Milanese Stuffed Zucchini

Placed sliced zucchini and water in a casserole. Microwave at full power for 3 minutes. Set apart. Microwave beef and onion at full power for 50 seconds, stirring twice. Add tomato, oregano, salt and pepper. Drain cooked zucchini and deposit in plate. Add meat and blend. Sprinkle with cheese and microwave at full power for 1 ½ minute. Let stand 3 minutes before serving. Makes 1 serving.

Beef, lean ground	3 oz (90 g)
Zucchini, sliced	⅔ cup (160 ml)
Onion, chopped	1 tbsp (15 ml)
Low fat mozzarella cheese, grated	1 tbsp (15 ml)
Garlic clove, chopped	1
Tomato (canned)	1
Water	¼ cup (60 ml)
Oregano	½ tsp (2 ml)
Salt and black pepper, to taste	

For one serving:

Carbohydrates: 17 g = 4 units
Fat: 16 g = 3 units
Proteins: 24 g
Calories: 300

❖

Stuffed Pepper, traditional oven

Cut off the top of the green pepper. In salted boiling water, blanche green pepper for 10 minutes. Drain and chill. Combine onion with ground beef, salt, pepper and chopped parsley. Stuff green pepper with beef mixture and place it in a baking dish. Pour tomato juice around and bake at 350 °F/180 °C for 1 hour. Serve. Makes 1 serving.

Green pepper	1
Onion, chopped	1 small
Beef, lean ground	4 oz (120 g)
Tomato juice	½ cup (125 ml)
Parsley, chopped	
Salt and black pepper	

For one serving:	
Carbohydrates:	28 g = 7 units
Fat:	18 g = 3.5 units
Proteins:	25 g
Calories:	361

❖

Stuffed Pepper with Cheese

Cut the green pepper in half, lengthwise. Blanch peppers in boiling water for 3 minutes; drain and set aside. Mix cottage cheese, rice, ketchup, Worcestershire sauce and seasonings. Stuff green peppers with this mixture. Sprinkle with grated cheese and bake at 375 °F/190 °C for 12 minutes. Makes 2 servings.

Green pepper	2 medium
Cottage cheese, 1 %	1 cup (250 ml)
Rice, cooked	½ cup (125 ml)
Ketchup	1 tbsp (15 ml)
Worcestershire sauce	½ tsp (2 ml)
Oregano	¼ tsp (1 ml)
Parmesan cheese, grated	1 tbsp (15 ml)
Salt and black pepper, to taste	

For one serving:
Carbohydrates: 24 g = 6 units
Fat: 2 g = 0.5 unit
Proteins: 10 g
Calories: 202

❖

Stuffed Green Pepper, microwave

Place onion and ground beef in microwave-safe dish. Microwave at full power for 1 ½ minute. Halve green pepper lengthwise, wash, core and discard stem. Place crushed tomato and bay leaf on a plate. Cover with green pepper halves. Fill peppers with meat, curry, tomato juice, onion and pepper. Microwave at full power for 6 minutes. Let stand 4 minutes before serving. Makes 1 serving.

Green pepper	1
Beef, lean ground	4 oz (120 g)
Tomato juice	1 tbsp (15 ml)
Tomato, fresh	1
Onion, chopped	1 tbsp (15 ml)
Curry	½ tsp (2 ml)
Bay leaf	1
Black pepper	

For one serving:

Carbohydrates:	7 g = 2 units
Fat:	17 g = 2.5 units
Proteins:	22 g
Calories:	273

❖

Roasted Peppers

Place peppers on the grill or under the oven broiler. Char peppers until blackened on all sides, turning as needed. The skin of the peppers will blister. Remove peppers and put in a bowl. Cover with plastic wrap and allow to cool. Peel skin from peppers and slice into thin strips. Peppers can be used in salads, puréed and thinned with chicken broth and heated as soup, or puréed and thinned with balsamic vinegar as salad dressing. Makes 6 servings.

Red pepper, whole	4
Yellow pepper, whole	4
Green pepper, whole	4

For one serving:
Carbohydrates: 14 g = 3.5 units
Fat: Trace amount
Proteins: 2 g
Calories: 60

❖

Spinach and Lemon

Wash and dry spinach. Steam for two or three minutes. Mix with lemon juice, broth and salt. Pour over spinach. Makes 4 servings.

Spinach	1 lb (454 g)
Lemon juice	1 tbsp (15 ml)
Chicken broth, fat free	3 tbsp (45 ml)
Sugar substitute	1 packet
Salt, to taste	

For one serving:
Carbohydrates: 3 g = 1 unit
Fat: Trace amount
Proteins: 2 g
Calories: 18

Spinach Gourmet

Cook spinach and drain well. In a Pam-sprayed casserole, mix all ingredients and cover. Cook one hour at 350 °F/180 °C. Makes 4 servings.

Spinach, chopped	4 cups (1 liter)
Fresh mushrooms	1 cup (250 ml)
Onion minced	2 tsp (10 ml)
Garlic clove minced	1
Mayonnaise, light	½ cup (125 ml)
Lemon juice	2 tbsp (30 ml)
Tabasco sauce, to taste	
Salt	1 tsp (5 ml)
Black pepper	1 pinch

For one serving:

Carbohydrates:	8 g = 2 units
Fat:	15 g = 3 units
Proteins:	1 g
Calories:	170

❖

Spinach Casserole

Cook the spinach and drain well. Combine eggs, onion and pepper. Add cheese and spinach. Pour into a casserole sprayed with Pam. Bake uncovered at 350 °F/180 °C for 15 minutes. Makes 1 serving.

Spinach	1 cup (250 ml)
Eggs (beaten)	2
Cheddar cheese, shredded	2 oz (60 g)
Onion, minced	1 tsp (5 ml)
Black pepper, to taste	

For one serving:

Carbohydrates:	3 g = 1 unit
Fat:	14 g = 3 units
Proteins:	27 g
Calories:	251

Spinach Soufflé

Blend all ingredients together, except spinach, in a food processor. Then, add spinach (thawed) and combine with egg mixture. Spray a baking dish with Pam and bake at 350 °F/ 180 °C for approximately 30 minutes. Good hot or cold. Makes 1 serving.

Eggs	2
Nutmeg	1 tsp (5 ml)
Spinach, frozen	1 cup (250 ml)
Vanilla	1 tsp (5 ml)
Sugar substitute	1 pouch

For one serving:

Carbohydrates:	2 g = 0.5 unit
Fat:	10 g = 2 units
Proteins:	13 g
Calories:	164

❖

Mushroom Snacks

Place mushrooms on Pam-sprayed cookie sheet and sprinkle with salt. Bake at 250 °F (120 °C) for 40-50 minutes until crispy. Eat like popcorn. Makes 2 servings.

Fresh mushrooms	1 lb (454 g)
Salt, to taste	

For one serving:

Carbohydrates:	10 g = 2 units
Fat:	Trace amount
Proteins:	4 g
Calories:	58

Baked Stuffed Mushrooms Florentine

Wash mushrooms, remove stems and chop, reserving caps. Combine all ingredients and spoon into caps. Put in baking dish sprayed with Pam and bake at 350 °F/180 °C for 15-20 minutes. One cup makes 1 serving.

Fresh mushrooms	1 lb (454 g)
Spinach, chopped	1 cup (250 ml)
Onion, minced	2 tsp (10 ml)
Chives	1 tsp (5 ml)
Thyme, fresh	1 tsp (5 ml)
Lemon juice	1 tbsp (15 ml)

For one serving:

Carbohydrates:	25 g = 2 units
Fat:	2 g = 1 unit
Proteins:	10 g
Calories:	128

❖

Mushroom Delight

Dice mushroom stems into small pieces. Combine seasonings and butter. Melt in microwave. Brush caps with melted butter and put in a casserole. Microwave on high for 8-10 minutes and set aside. Rinse crabmeat and mix with cheese and mushroom stems. Microwave mixture on high 3-4 minutes. Stir well and divide mixture into mushroom caps. Microwave on high for 3 minutes; sprinkle with lemon juice and paprika. Serve while hot. Makes 2 servings.

Fresh mushrooms	8 large
Canned crab	8 oz (240 g)
Cheddar cheese 7 %, grated	4 oz (120 g)
Butter	2 tsp (10 ml)
Lemon juice	½ tsp (2 ml)
Paprika, to taste	
Salt and pepper, to taste	

For one serving:

Carbohydrates:	6 g = 1.5 units
Fat:	8 g = 1.5 units
Proteins:	33 g
Calories:	226

❖

Broccoli or Cauliflower in Tomato Sauce

Steam broccoli or cauliflower. Heat tomatoes, oil, vinegar and oregano. Pour over hot, drained vegetables. Sprinkle with light salt, if needed. Makes 2 to 4 servings.

Broccoli or cauliflower	10 oz (300 g)
Tomatoes, crushed	½ cup (125 ml)
Vinegar balsamic	1 ½ tsp (2 ml)
Oregano	¼ tsp (1 ml)
Garlic, chopped	1 clove
Basil	½ tsp (2 ml)
Chili powder, to taste	
Salt to taste	

For one serving:
Carbohydrates: 9 g = 2 units
Fat: Trace amount
Proteins: 4 g
Calories: 48

❖

Caraway Cabbage

Cook cabbage in boiling water, salt and sweetener for 5 minutes. Cover and cook until cabbage is tender, about 3 minutes. Drain, stir in remaining ingredients. Makes 2 servings.

Cabbage, shredded	2 cups (500 ml)
Water (hot)	½ cup (125 ml)
Salt	½ tsp (2 ml)
Sugar substitute	1 tsp (5 ml)
Onion minced	1 tsp (5 ml)
Marjoram	¾ tsp (4 ml)
Curry seeds	½ tsp (2 ml)
Black pepper	⅛ tsp (0.5 ml)

For one serving:

Carbohydrates:	12 g = 3 units
Fat:	Trace amount
Proteins:	3 g
Calories:	55

❖

Stuffed Cabbage

Microwave the cabbage at full power for 2 minutes. Meanwhile, mix meat, shallot, pepper and half the quantity of tomato juice. Make 2 rolls with meat and cabbage leaves. Place the 2 rolls in a baking dish. Microwave at full power for 5 minutes. Let stand 3 minutes before serving. Makes 1 serving.

Cabbage	2 leaves
Beef, lean ground	4 oz (120 g)
Shallot, chopped	2 tbsp (30 ml)
Tomato juice	2 tbsp (30 ml)
Consommé (onion), fat free	¼ cup (60 ml)
Black pepper, to taste	

For one serving:	
Carbohydrates:	8 g = 2 units
Fat:	17 g = 3.5 units
Proteins:	22 g
Calories:	276

❖

Cauliflower and Artichoke

Steam the cauliflower, add the remaining vegetables and curry and marinate in refrigerator. Makes 4 servings.

Cauliflower	2 cups (500 ml)
Artichoke	1 cup (250 ml)
Fresh mushrooms	4 oz (120 g)
Shallot	4
Olive oil	2 tbsp (30 ml)
Wine vinegar	1 tbsp (15 ml)
Dijon mustard	1 tbsp (15 ml)

For one serving:	
Carbohydrates:	12 g = 3 units
Fat:	3 g = 0.5 unit
Proteins:	4 g
Calories:	76

Tasty Red Cabbage

Put all ingredients in a pot and simmer for 30 minutes. Drain cabbage and serve. Makes 3 servings.

Cabbage (red)	2 cups (500 ml)
Apple, quartered	½
Onion, quartered	1
Water	½ cup (125 ml)
Apple cider vinegar	1 tsp (5 ml)
Salt	½ tsp (2 ml)

For one serving:

Carbohydrates:	80 g = 20 units
Fat:	4 g = 1 unit
Proteins:	18 g
Calories:	347

❖

Stir-fried Cabbage

Combine sugar substitute, vinegar, soy sauce, pepper and salt. Heat 1 tbsp of oil in wok or large skillet, add garlic and green onions and stir-fry 2-3 minutes. Stir in the vinegar mixture and cabbage and heat thoroughly. Makes 4 servings.

Cabbage, thinly sliced	4 cups (1 liter)
Sugar substitute	½ tsp (2 ml)
White vinegar	2 tbsp (30 ml)
Vegetable oil	1 tsp (5 ml)

SAUCE:	
Soy sauce, sugar free	2 tbsp (30 ml)
Garlic clove, minced	2
Onion, chopped	1 cup (250 ml)
Ginger, minced	2 tbsp (30 ml)
Salt and pepper	½ tsp (2 ml)

For one serving:

Carbohydrates:	17 g = 4 units
Fat:	4 g = 1 unit
Proteins:	4 g
Calories:	115

❖

Bean Sprouts with Italian Rice

In a skillet, sauté all the vegetables on medium heat for 5 minutes. Season. Combine the vegetables, cooked beans, cooked rice and cheese and mix well. Heat on low until the cheese melts. Add chopped parsley and mix. Makes 2 servings.

Olive oil	1 tsp (5 ml)
Broccoli, cubed	¾ cup (180 ml)
Carrot, strips	¼ cup (60 ml)
Fresh celery, cut	½ cup (125 ml)
Tomato, sliced	1
Garlic clove, chopped	1
Basil	½ tsp (2 ml)
Oregano	½ tsp (2 ml)
Bean sprouts, cooked	½ cup (125 ml)
Rice, cooked brown	½ cup (125 ml)
Low fat mozzarella cheese, grated	¼ cup (60 ml)
Parsley (fresh), chopped	2 tbsp (30 ml)
Salt	½ tsp (2 ml)

For one serving:

Carbohydrates:	28 g = 7 units
Fat:	10 g = 2 units
Proteins:	17 g
Calories:	256

❖

Bean Sprouts, Alfalfa and Spinach

Thoroughly wash spinach and cut off the stems. Shred spinach into pieces and mix with other ingredients. Top with vinaigrette. Makes 4 servings.

Spinach	10 oz (300 g)
Bean sprouts	2 cups (500 ml)
Alfalfa	1 cup (250 ml)
Hard boiled eggs, sliced	4
Choice of vinaigrette, low-fat	¼ cup (60 ml)

For one serving:

Carbohydrates:	7 g = 2 units
Fat:	6 g = 1 unit
Proteins:	9 g
Calories:	115

❖

Tangy Green Beans

Heat salt, sweetener and oil. Add beans, heat thoroughly. Then add lemon juice and vinegar right before serving. Makes 3 servings.

Green beans, cooked	3 cup (750 ml)
Lemon juice	2 tbsp (30 ml)
Vinegar	2 tbsp (30 ml)
Olive oil	2 tsp (10 ml)
Mustard powder	1 tbsp (15 ml)
Sugar substitute (liquid)	¾ tsp (4 ml)
Salt	½ tsp (2 ml)

For one serving:

Carbohydrates:	9 g = 2 units
Fat:	3 g = 1 unit
Proteins:	2 g
Calories:	67

Tangy Mustard Beans

Place beans, water and salt in medium size sauce pan. Cover and bring to boil over moderately high heat. Reduce heat and cook about 15 minutes. Mix remaining ingredients in small bowl, pour over undrained beans and stir to completely coat. Leftovers are delicious cold. Makes 4 servings.

Green beans	1 lb (454 g)
Mustard (Dijon)	2 tsp (10 ml)
Olive oil	2 tsp (10 ml)
Vinegar (white)	3 tbsp (45 ml)
Sugar substitute	½ tsp (2 ml)
Water to cover beans	
Salt	¾ tsp (4 ml)

For one serving:
Carbohydrates: 8 g = 2 units
Fat: 3 g = 0.5 unit
Proteins: 2 g
Calories: 60

❖

Tasty Green Beans

Place all ingredients in a sauce pan. Bring to rapid boil. Reduce heat to simmer for 3-5 minutes. Makes 1 serving.

Green beans	3 ½ oz (105 g)
Chicken broth, fat free	½ cup (125 ml)
Fresh celery, chopped	2 tsp (10 ml)
Onion, minced	1 tsp (5 ml)
Water	½ cup (125 ml)

For one serving:
Carbohydrates: 9 g = 2 units
Fat: 0
Proteins: 2 g
Calories: 41

Tuna-Stuffed Tomato

Wash the tomato and cut off top. Core tomato and drain before filling. Combine all ingredients and fill the tomato. Serve tomato on lettuce leaf and garnish with fresh parsley. Makes 1 serving.

Tomato	1 medium
Tuna	3 oz (90 g)
Fresh celery, cubed	2 tbsp (30 ml)
Onion chopped	1 tbsp (15 ml)
Plain yogurt, 2 %	1 tsp (5 ml)
Lettuce	1 leaf
Parsley, to taste	
Salt, to taste	
Black pepper, to taste	

For one serving:

Carbohydrates:	8 g	= 2 units
Fat:	3 g	= 0.5 unit
Proteins:	21 g	
Calories:	145	

❖

Broiled Tomato

Cut tomato in half and sprinkle with sweetener and cinnamon. Broil and eat. Makes 1 serving.

Tomato	1
Sugar substitute	1 pouch
Cinnamon, to taste	

> **For one serving:**
> Carbohydrates: 6 g = 1.5 units
> Fat: 0
> Proteins: 1 g
> Calories: 26

❖

Super Tomatoes

Peel tomatoes by immersing them in hot water until peels begin to split. Put in cold water immediately to cool. Skins will pull off easily. Slice tomatoes into ½ inch (1 cm) thick slices. Season lightly with salt and freshly ground pepper, basil leaves, lime juice, sugar and garlic mixed with olive oil. Allow to stand, covered, at least 15 minutes, before serving. Makes 4 servings.

Tomatoes	4
Basil, chopped	6 leaves
Lemon juice	1 tsp (5 ml)
Sugar substitute	½ tsp (2 ml)
Garlic clove, minced	1
Olive oil	1 tbsp (15 ml)
Salt, to taste	
Black pepper, to taste	

> **For one serving:**
> Carbohydrates: 2 g = 0.5 unit
> Fat: 3 g = 0.5 unit
> Proteins: Trace amount
> Calories: 39

Stuffed Cucumber

Wash and cut cucumber in half, lengthwise. Spoon out center seeds. Finely dice onion, radishes, celery, and lettuce. Add seasonings. Add vinegar and oil. Blend together well and spoon into the cucumber boats. Serve on Romaine leaf. Top with mushroom caps. Makes 1 serving.

Cucumber	1 medium
Onion	⅛ cup (30 ml)
Radishes	⅛ cup (30 ml)
Fresh celery	⅛ cup (30 ml)
Lettuce	⅛ cup (30 ml)
White wine vinegar	1 tbsp (15 ml)
Olive oil	1 tbsp (15 ml)
Garlic, minced	½ tsp (2 ml)
Dill seeds	1 pinch
Romaine lettuce	1 leaf
Fresh mushrooms	3

For one serving:

Carbohydrates:	17 g = 4 units
Fat:	14 g = 3 units
Proteins:	5 g
Calories:	207

❖

Stir-Fry

Heat oil in large skillet. Stir-fry zucchini, onion, ginger and garlic until vegetables are tender-crisp, about 5 min. Mix soy sauce, tabasco and water. Add to skillet along with tomatoes and cook one more minute. Makes 2 servings.

Vegetable oil	1 tbsp (15 ml)
Zucchini, sliced	½ lb (227 g)
Onion, minced	1
Ginger fresh root	1 tsp (5 ml)
Garlic clove, chopped	1
Soy sauce, sugar free	1 tbsp (15 ml)
Tabasco sauce	¼ tsp (1 ml)
Water	⅓ cup (80 ml)
Tomatoes (cherry)	1 cup (250 ml)

For one serving:

Carbohydrates:	15 g = 4 units
Fat:	6 g = 1 unit
Proteins:	8 g
Calories:	133

❖

Gazpacho

Dissolve broth in water, and add other ingredients in given order. Blend. Chill for 3 or 4 hours. Makes 4 servings.

Water (hot)	2 cups (500 ml)
Chicken broth, fat free	2 tsp (10 ml)
Tomatoes, pured	2 cups (500 ml)
Black pepper	½ tsp (2 ml)
Cucumber, cubed	1
Onion, chopped	½ cup (125 ml)
Green pepper	½

For one serving:

Carbohydrates:	14 g = 3.5 units
Fat:	Trace amount
Proteins:	2 g
Calories:	60

❖

Molded Garden Relish

Pour boiling water over gelatin in bowl, stirring until dissolved. Chill until slightly thickened. Stir in cucumber, celery, onion flakes and salt. Chill until firm and unmold on celery leaves. Makes 4 to 6 servings.

Gelatin (unflavored)	2 envelopes
Water, boiling	1 ½ cup (375 ml)
Cucumber, pared and shredded	1 cup (250 ml)
Fresh celery, thinly sliced	1 cup (250 ml)
Onion, chopped	¼ cup (60 ml)
Sugar substitute	½ tsp (2 ml)
Fresh celery leaves	
Salt	2 tsp (10 ml)

For one serving:

Carbohydrates:	19 g = 5 units
Fat:	1 g
Proteins:	16 g
Calories:	135

❖

Garden Vegetable Casserole

Place all sliced vegetables in a pan and mix all other ingredients. Place in oven for 20-25 minutes at 350 °F/180 °C. Makes 4 servings.

May be cooked in microwave for 8 to 10 minutes.

Squash, sliced	2
Parmesan Cheese, grated	2 tsp (10 ml)
Zucchini, sliced	1 medium
Onion, sliced	1 small
Tomato, sliced	1
Basil	½ tsp (2 ml)
Thyme	½ tsp (2 ml)
Salt	½ tsp (2 ml)

For one serving:
Carbohydrates: 10 g = 2.5 units
Fat: Trace amount
Proteins: 3 g
Calories: 50

Baked Mixed Vegetables

Put all ingredients into casserole and bake uncovered at 350 °F/180 °C for 30 minutes. Makes 2 servings.

Green beans	1 cup (250 ml)
Tomatoes, chopped	½ cup (125 ml)
Fresh celery, cut into strips	½ cup (125 ml)
Green pepper, cut into strips	½ cup (125 ml)
Onion, cut into strips	¼ cup (60 ml)
Olive oil	3 tbsp (45 ml)
Salt	¾ tsp (4 ml)

For one serving:
Carbohydrates: 13 g = 3 units
Fat: 21 g = 5 units
Proteins: 2 g
Calories: 254

❖

Rice Loaf with Carrot

Combine all ingredients and put them in a baking dish. Bake at 325 °F/160 °C for about 30 minutes. Makes 2 servings.

Rice, cooked	½ cup (125 ml)
Egg, beaten	1
Carrot, grated	¾ cup (180 ml)
Cheddar cheese, grated	½ cup (125 ml)
Worcestershire sauce	½ tsp (2 ml)
Mustard, dried	½ tsp (2 ml)
Salt	¼ tsp (1 ml)
Black pepper	1 pinch

For one serving:
Carbohydrates: 25 g = 6 units
Fat: 7 g = 1.5 units
Proteins: 22 g
Calories: 257

Legume Loaf

Squash chick peas. Add all other ingredients and mix well. Put in a small greased baking dish. Bake at 350 °F/180 °C for about 30 minutes. Serve with tomato sauce. Makes 2 servings.

Chick peas (canned)	¾ cup (180 ml)
Onion, chopped	2 tbsp (30 ml)
Fresh celery, chopped	2 tbsp (30 ml)
Green pepper, chopped	¼ cup (60 ml)
Carrot, grated	2 tbsp (30 ml)
Egg (beaten)	1
Low fat cheese, grated	½ cup (125 ml)
Oatmeal	2 tbsp (30 ml)
Parsley (fresh), chopped	1 tbsp (15 ml)
Basil	3 leaves
Soy sauce, sugar free	½ tsp (2 ml)
Garlic clove, chopped	1
Worcestershire sauce	½ tsp (2 ml)

For one serving:

Carbohydrates: 42 g = 10 units
Fat: 10 g = 2 units
Proteins: 26 g
Calories: 358

❖

Ratatouille Niçoise

Place eggplant and onion in baking dish and microwave at full power for 1 minute. Add zucchini, garlic, green pepper and tomato paste. Cover and microwave at full power for 1 minute. Add remaining ingredients and microwave at full power for 1 minute. Serve warm. Makes 1 serving.

Eggplant, peeled and cubed	2 cups (500 ml)
Zucchini, sliced	1
Tomato, peeled and cubed	1
Garlic clove, chopped	1
Green pepper strips	½ cup (125 ml)
Onion, minced	2 tbsp (30 ml)
Tomato paste	½ tsp (2 ml)
Basil	¼ tsp (1 ml)
Parsley, chopped, to taste	
Oregano	¼ tsp (1 ml)
Salt and black pepper, to taste	

For one serving:	
Carbohydrates:	35 g = 9 units
Fat:	1 g
Proteins:	6 g
Calories:	154

❖

Soup Supreme

Place all ingredients in a food processor and mix well. Heat and serve. Makes 1 serving.

Asparagus, with liquid	¾ cup (180 ml)
Chicken broth, fat free	1 cup (250 ml)
Onion, chopped	½ tsp (2 ml)
Chives	½ tsp (2 ml)
Butter	½ tsp (2 ml)
Black pepper, to taste	

For one serving:

Carbohydrates: 5 g = 1 unit
Fat: 3 g = 0.5 unit
Proteins: 4 g
Calories: 52

❖

Mock Sour Cream Dip

Process all ingredients in blender until smooth. Makes 4 servings.

Sour cream, 14 %	1 cup (250 ml)
Mayonnaise, light	¼ cup (60 ml)
Lemon juice	2 tbsp (30 ml)
Paprika, to taste	
Dill, fresh	2 tsp (10 ml)
Onion, chopped	1 tbsp (15 ml)
Garlic clove, chopped	1

For one serving:

Carbohydrates: 5 g = 1 unit
Fat: 13 g = 2.5 units
Proteins: 2 g
Calories: 143

Cheese Dip

Process all ingredients in food processor until smooth. Cover and chill. (Dip any fresh vegetables into this mix). Makes 2 servings.

Cottage cheese, skimmed	½ cup (125 ml)
Cheddar cheese, sharp, grated	¼ cup (60 ml)
Dill fresh, to taste	

For one serving:
Carbohydrates: 2 g = 0.5 unit
Fat: 10 g = 2 units
Proteins: 15 g
Calories: 165

---------- ❖ ----------

Eggs and Vegetables Salad

Steam cauliflower until a little more than "crispy", cool and break into flowerets. Combine the rest of ingredients and add cauliflower. Mix well, add parsley flakes and sprinkle with paprika. Makes 2 servings.

Cauliflower	1
Cucumber, chopped	¼ cup (60 ml)
Fresh celery	¼ cup (60 ml)
Eggs (hard boiled), chopped	2
Onion, minced, to taste	
Paprika	¼ tsp (1 ml)
Red pepper, chopped	2 tbsp (30 ml)
Mayonnaise, light	2 tbsp (30 ml)
Salt and pepper, to taste	

For one serving:
Carbohydrates: 8 g = 2 units
Fat: 10 g = 2 units
Proteins: 8 g
Calories: 150

Spiced Pear Salad

Combine pear juice, vinegar, cinnamon stick, and clove. Bring to boil and cook 2 minutes. Pour hot mixture over pears and chill several hours. Arrange pears on bol of lettuce and combine juice with mayonnaise and serve over pears. Makes 4 servings.

Pear halves (canned)	2 cans
Vinegar, red wine	1 tbsp (15 ml)
Cinnamon stick	1
Clove	1
Lettuce, shredded	1 cup (250 ml)
Mayonnaise, light	1 tbsp (15 ml)

For one serving:
Carbohydrates: 25 g = 6 units
Fat: 2 g = 0.5 unit
Proteins: 2 g
Calories: 115

❖

Egg and Cottage Salad

Cut egg in two: keep half of egg yolk for garnish. Cut egg into small pieces. Add the rest of the ingredients. Mix well and serve on a bed of lettuce. Place the yolk on the salad. Garnish with parsley. Makes 1 serving.

Egg, hard boiled	1
Cottage Cheese	3 tbsp (45 ml)
Plain yogurt, 2 %	1 tbsp (15 ml)
Shallot, finely chopped	1 ½ tsp (7 ml)
Worcestershire sauce	4-5 drops
Lettuce leaf	1
Parsley	
Salt and pepper, to taste	

For one serving:

Carbohydrates:	4 g = 1 unit
Fat:	6 g = 1 unit
Proteins:	13 g
Calories:	121

❖

Hot Salmon and Cabbage Salad

Drain salmon and break it in chunks. Stir-fry cabbage and carrot in oil 5 minutes or until tender crisp, stir frequently. Sprinkle with vinegar, sugar, celery seed and salt. Add salmon and toss. Reheat 3 to 5 minutes. Remove from heat. Fold in parsley, yogurt and salad dressing. Makes 2 servings.

Salmon, canned	6 oz (180 g)
Vegetable oil	2 tsp (10 ml)
Cabbage, thinly shredded	2 cups (500 ml)
Carrot, grated	⅓ cup (80 ml)
Vinegar	1 tbsp (15 ml)
Sugar substitute	½ tsp (2 ml)
Celery seeds	¼ tsp (1 ml)
Parsley, chopped	1 tbsp (15 ml)
Plain yogurt, 2 %	2 tbsp (30 ml)
Salad dressing, light	1 tbsp (15 ml)
Salt	1 pinch

For one serving:
Carbohydrates: 16 g = 4 units
Fat: 11 g = 2 units
Proteins: 22 g
Calories: 245

❖

Asparagus Tips

Cook asparagus in boiling water until barely tender. Drain and chill. Combine onion, pepper, mustard, oil, white vinegar and chill. Pour over asparagus just before serving. Makes 4 servings.

Asparagus	24 tips
Water, boiling	8 cups (2 liters)
Onion, minced	1 tsp (5 ml)
Mustard, prepared	¼ tsp (1 ml)
Olive oil	1 tbsp (15 ml)
White vinegar	2 tbsp (30 ml)
Black pepper, to taste	

For one serving:
Carbohydrates: 3 g = 1 unit
Fat: 4 g = 1 unit
Proteins: 2 g
Calories: 51

❖

Cucumber Salad

Mix and chill covered at least 2 hours. After, add 1 cup of mayonnaise for each cup of the fresh vegetable mixture.

Cucumber, sliced	4
Radishes, chopped	4
Fresh mushrooms, chopped	4
Cauliflower, chopped	1 cup (250 ml)
Onion, green, chopped	2
Mayonnaise, light	1 tbsp (15 ml)
Dijon mustard	1 tsp (5 ml)

For one serving:
Carbohydrates: 13 g = 2.5 units
Fat: 1 g
Proteins: 4 g
Calories: 74

Zucchini Slaw

Dilute the mayonnaise with 2 tsp of water and mix until smooth. Add 4 drops of sweetener and the celery seeds. Toss dressing and vegetables together. Chill. Makes 2 servings.

Zucchini, shredded	2 cups (500 ml)
Raisins	4 tbsp (60 ml)
Mayonnaise, light	2 tbsp (30 ml)
Celery seeds	1 pinch
Water	2 tsp (10 ml)
Sugar substitute, a few drops	

For one serving:

Carbohydrates:	25 g = 6 units
Fat:	5 g = 1 unit
Proteins:	4 g
Calories:	146

❖

Crab Salad

Mix crab meat, apple and green pepper. Mix mayonnaise, yogurt, lemon juice and curry powder. Add to crab mixture. Refrigerate until ready to serve. Arrange on a bed of lettuce, garnish with parsley and half a lemon slice. Makes 2 servings.

Crab (canned)	6 oz (180 g)
Apple (unpeeled), cubes	1
Green pepper	½
Mayonnaise, light	1 tsp (5 ml)
Plain yogurt, 2 %	1 tsp (5 ml)
Curry powder	1 ½ tsp (7 ml)
Lettuce leaves	2
Lemon, sliced	1
Parsley, to taste	
Lemon juice	1 tsp (5 ml)

For one serving:

Carbohydrates:	13 g = 3 units
Fat:	2 g = 0.5 unit
Proteins:	18 g
Calories:	144

❖

Hot Crab Salad

Heat oven to 400 °F/205 °C. Mix all ingredients together and put in a Pam-sprayed baking dish. Bake uncovered 10 minutes, or until thoroughly heated. Makes 3 servings.

Canned crab	1 cup (250 ml)
Fresh celery	⅓ cup (80 ml)
Eggs, cooked, chopped	3
Onion, chopped	2 tbsp (30 ml)
Mayonnaise, light	¼ cup (60 ml)
Lemon juice	1 tsp (5 ml)
Salt and black pepper, to taste	

For one serving:

Carbohydrates:	4 g = 1 unit
Fat:	9 g = 2 units
Proteins:	16 g
Calories:	160

❖

Tasty Shrimp Salad

Cut green peppers crosswise in half; remove seeds and membranes. Wash insides and outsides and pat dry. Drain shrimp, rinse in cold water and drain again. Mix with remaining ingredients and spoon salad into pepper shells. Makes 4 servings.

Green pepper	4
Fresh celery, chopped	1 cup (250 ml)
Shrimp, cooked	1 lb (454 g)
Mayonnaise, light	1 cup (250 ml)
Onion, minced	2 tbsp (30 ml)
Vinegar (white)	2 tbsp (30 ml)
Salt and black pepper, to taste	

For one serving:
Carbohydrates: 10 g = 2.5 units
Fat: 11 g = 2 units
Proteins: 25 g
Calories: 245

❖

Chicken or Turkey Salad

Toss chicken, celery, green pepper, onion and mayonnaise.
Cover and chill. Serve on spinach leaves. Garnish salad with
lemon wedge. Makes 2 servings.

Chicken or turkey, cubed	1 cup (250 ml)
Fresh celery, chopped	¾ cup (180 ml)
Green pepper, diced	¾ cup (180 ml)
Onion, chopped	3 tbsp (45 ml)
Mayonnaise, light	¼ cup (60 ml)
Spinach leaves	1 cup (250 ml)
Lemon, few drops	

For one serving:

Carbohydrates:	8 g = 2 units
Fat:	22 g = 4.5 units
Proteins:	22 g
Calories:	321

❖

Hot Spinach Salad

Remove stems from spinach, wash leaves and drain. Put in a large steamer (in a saucepan without water), cover and steam 2-3 minutes, or just until leaves wilt; drain any liquid from pan. Combine lemon juice, broth and artificial sweetener, pour over spinach and toss. Makes 2 servings.

Spinach	2 cups (500 ml)
Lemon juice	1 tsp (5 ml)
Chicken broth, fat free	3 tbsp (45 ml)
Sugar substitute	1 tsp (5 ml)
Worcestershire sauce	$\frac{1}{4}$ tsp (1 ml)
Vegetable oil	1 tbsp (15 ml)

For one serving:
Carbohydrates: 1 g
Fat: 7 g = 1.5 units
Proteins: Trace amount
Calories: 62

❖

Ceasar Salad

Just before serving, rub large salad bowl with cut garlic clove. Add oil, salt, pepper and mix thoroughly. Into a bowl, tear spinach into bite size pieces and toss until leaves glisten. Break egg into spinach. Squeeze on juice from lemon; toss until leaves are well coated. Makes 8 servings.

Garlic clove, halved	1
Olive oil	½ cup (125 ml)
Spinach	1 package of 10 oz (300 g)
Egg	1
Lemon juice	1 tsp (5 ml)
Mustard (Dijon)	1 tsp (5 ml)
Salt	1 tsp (5 ml)
Black pepper, to taste	

For one serving:

Carbohydrates:	2 g = 0.5 unit
Fat:	14 = 3 units
Proteins:	Trace amount
Calories:	131

❖

Spinach-Sprout Salad

Combine spinach and sprouts. Mix oil, vinegar, chili powder, salt and pepper. Toss with spinach and sprouts and garnish with eggs. Makes 4 to 6 servings.

Egg (hard boiled), cut into quarters	1
Spinach	4-6 cups (1-1.5 liter)
Bean sprouts	3 cups (750 ml)
Vinegar (rice)	1 tbsp (15 ml)
Chili powder	2 tsp (10 ml)
Safflower oil	2 tbsp (30 ml)
Salt and black pepper, to taste	

For one serving:

Carbohydrates:	7 g = 2 units
Fat:	10 g = 2 units
Proteins:	9 g
Calories:	135

❖

Green Bean and Sprout Salad

Marinate all ingredients except sprouts in refrigerator 2 to 4 hours. Add bean sprouts, serve on spinach leaves. Makes 4 servings.

Fresh mushrooms, sliced	1 cup (250 ml)
Bean sprouts	2 cups (500 ml)
Safflower oil	1 tbsp (15 ml)
Vinegar (white)	2 tbsp (30 ml)
Garlic clove, chopped	1
Salt, to taste	
Black pepper, to taste	

For one serving:

Carbohydrates:	5 g = 1 unit
Fat:	4 g = 1 unit
Proteins:	2 g
Calories:	80

❖

Tangy Wilted Spinach Salad

Wash spinach and remove stems; dry leaves. Tear leaves into bite-size pieces. In a small saucepan, heat sugar substitute, vinegar, water, salad oil, salt, dill weed, mustard and pepper to boiling. Pour over greens and toss. Makes 6 servings.

Spinach	½ lb (225 g)
Sugar substitute	½ tsp (2 ml)
Vinegar (white)	¼ cup (60 ml)
Water	2 tbsp (30 ml)
Olive oil	2 tbsp (30 ml)
Dill	½ tsp (2 ml)
Mustard (dry)	½ tsp (2 ml)
Salt and black pepper, to taste	

For one serving:

Carbohydrates:	2 g = 0.5 unit
Fat:	5 g = 1 unit
Proteins:	Trace amount
Calories:	47

❖

Chicken Salad

In a medium-sized bowl, pour lemon juice over chicken. Add remaining ingredients, toss and serve on crisp leaves, or in green pepper rings. Makes 6 servings.

Lemon juice	3 tbsp (45 ml)
Chicken, cooked, diced	4 cups (1 liter)
Fresh celery, chopped	1 cup (250 ml)
Onion, minced	⅓ cup (80 ml)
Mayonnaise, light	⅓ cup (80 ml)
Red pepper a few slices	
Salt and pepper, to taste	

For one serving:

Carbohydrates:	5 g = 1 unit
Fat:	12 g = 2.5 units
Proteins:	10 g
Calories:	161

———— ❖ ————

Chicken Zucchini Salad

Combine chicken, zucchini, mayonnaise and onion. Arrange on lettuce leaf. Arrange tomato wedges around salad. Makes 1 serving.

Chicken (cooked), cubes	4 oz (120 g)
Zucchini, minced	½ cup (125 ml)
Mayonnaise, light	1 tbsp (15 ml)
Onion, minced	1 tbsp (15 ml)
Tomato in quarters	1
Lettuce leaves	

For one serving:

Carbohydrates:	11 g = 3 units
Fat:	19 g = 5 units
Proteins:	27 g
Calories:	322

Chicken and Egg Salad

Combine and serve on lettuce leaf. Makes 1 serving.

Chicken cooked, chopped	4 oz (120 g)
Eggs (boiled), mashed	1
Mayonnaise, light	1 tbsp (15 ml)
Salt and black pepper, to taste	

For one serving:

Carbohydrates:	2 g = 0.5 unit
Fat:	21 g = 4 units
Proteins:	29 g
Calories:	308

❖

Confetti Salad

Combine first 5 ingredients in a bowl. Thoroughly mix other ingredients in another bowl, and pour over vegetables. Marinate at least 2 hours before serving. Makes 4 servings.

Green pepper, thinly sliced	1
Red pepper, thinly sliced	1
Shallot, chopped	2
Tomatoes in quarters	2
Cucumber, thinly sliced	2
Lemon juice	1 tbsp (15 ml)
Garlic powder	¼ tsp (1 ml)
Sugar substitute	½ tsp (2 ml)
Vegetable oil	2 tbsp (30 ml)
Black pepper	¼ tsp (1 ml)

For one serving:

Carbohydrates:	8 g = 2 units
Fat:	8 g = 2 units
Proteins:	1 g
Calories:	101

Hawaiian Salad

Wash, trim and chill salad greens. Chill salad plates, put pineapple into bowl, sprinkle with lemon juice, add sweetener if needed. Put in refrigerator to chill. Wash and pick over grapes or berries, slice in half over bowl to save any juice. Take pre-chilled greens, plates, and pineapple from fridge; place lettuce leaves on plates and heap pineapple into lettuce. Arrange grape or berry halves on pineapple. Garnish with watercress. Combine pineapple and berry or grape juice and use as salad dressing. Makes 4 servings.

Pineapple, diced	2 cups (500 ml)
Lemon juice	2 tbsp (30 ml)
Grapes or strawberries	1 lb (454 g)
Sugar substitute, to taste	
Lettuce	3-4 leaves
Watercress	1 bunch

For one serving:
Carbohydrates: 35 g = 9 units
Fat: 1 g
Proteins: 1 g
Calories: 136

❖

Perfection Salad

Mix together gelatin, sugar substitute and salt. Add boiling water and stir to completely dissolve gelatin. Add cold water, vinegar and lemon juice. Chill until partially set. Add remaining ingredients and pour into 8 x 8 x 2 inch pan (20 cm x 20 cm x 5 cm). Chill until firm. Makes 4 servings.

Gelatin (unflavored)	2 envelopes
Sugar substitute	1 envelope
Water (boiling)	1 ½ cup (375 ml)
Water (cold)	1 ½ cup (375 ml)
Vinegar (white)	½ cup (125 ml)
Lemon juice	2 tbsp (30 ml)
Alfalfa sprouts	2 cups (500 ml)
Fresh celery, chopped	1 cup (250 ml)
Radishes, chopped	¼ cup (60 ml)
Green pepper, chopped	¼ cup (60 ml)
Cucumber, sliced	½ cup (125 ml)
Salt	¼ tsp (1 ml)

For one serving:

Carbohydrates:	6 g = 1.5 units
Fat:	Trace amount
Proteins:	5 g
Calories:	43

❖

Spring Salad

Soften gelatin in cold water 5 minutes; dissolve in hot water. In a bowl, add lemon juice, vinegar and salt. Chill until partially set; add remaining ingredients. Pour into individual molds. Chill until firm. Serve on crisp spinach leaf and top with mayonnaise. Makes 4 servings.

Gelatin (unflavored)	1 pouch
Water (hot)	1 ¾ cup (430 ml)
Lemon juice	1 tbsp (15 ml)
White vinegar	1 tbsp (15 ml)
Cucumber, in cubes	1 cup (250 ml)
Fresh celery, chopped	1 cup (250 ml)
Red onion, chopped	⅓ cup (80 ml)
Radishes	½ cup (125 ml)
Salt	¼ tsp (1 ml)

For one serving:

Carbohydrates:	9 g = 2 units
Fat:	0
Proteins:	3 g
Calories:	54

❖

Beef Cannelloni

In non-stick pan, cook celery, garlic and mushrooms for 3 minutes. Set aside.

SAUCE:

Combine milk with seasonings and cook on low heat for 5 minutes. Add cornstarch mixed with water. Stir until it thickens. Take some of the sauce and mix it with the vegetables, beef and parmesan cheese. Stuff cannelloni with meat mixture and put in a baking dish sprayed with Pam. Top cannelloni with the remaining sauce and sprinkle with grated cheese. Cover and bake at 350 °F/180 °C for 10 minutes. Uncover and continue cooking for 2 more minutes. Garnish with parsley. Makes 2 servings.

Fresh celery, chopped	⅓ cup (80 ml)
Garlic clove, chopped	1
Fresh mushrooms, chopped	⅓ cup (80 ml)
Beef cooked ground	1 cup (250 ml)
Parmesan cheese, grated	1 tbsp (15 ml)
Cannelloni, cooked	4
Low fat mozzarella cheese, grated	¼ cup (60 ml)
Parsley, chopped (fresh)	1 tbsp (15 ml)
SAUCE:	
2 % partially skimmed milk	1 cup (250 ml)
Nutmeg	1 pinch
Cornstarch	2 tsp (10 ml)
Water cold	1 tbsp (15 ml)
Parsley, chopped (fresh)	1 tsp (5 ml)

For one serving:
Carbohydrates: 35 g = 9 units
Fat: 30 g = 6 units
Proteins: 57 g
Calories: 644

❖

Macaroni with Beef au Gratin

Cook pasta. In a non-stick pan, cook ground beef. Set aside. In the same pan, cook onions and garlic. Add mushrooms, remove beef and parsley, beef and cook for 5 minutes. Add tomatoes, season and let simmer for 15 minutes stirring often. Combine meat with pasta and put in a baking dish. Top with cheese and bake 20 to 25 minutes. Then grill cheese until it is browned. Makes 2 servings.

Beef, lean ground	8 oz (240 g)
Onion, chopped	½ cup (125 ml)
Fresh mushrooms, sliced	1 cup (250 ml)
Parsley, chopped	1 tbsp (15 ml)
Tomatoes, crushed	2 cups (500 ml)
Basil	¼ tsp (1 ml)
Oregano	¼ tsp (1 ml)
Low fat mozzarella cheese, grated	1 oz (30 g)
Macaroni, cooked	1 cup (250 ml)
Garlic, chopped	
Salt	¼ tsp (1 ml)
Black pepper	¼ tsp (1 ml)

For one serving:	
Carbohydrates:	30 g = 7.5 units
Fat:	20 g = 4 units
Proteins:	31 g
Calories:	425

❖

Manicotti with Salmon Sauce

Break salmon into small chunks and crush the bones. Carefully mix the salmon, bones, juice, celery soup, yogurt and parsley. In a non-stick pan, cook onion and garlic then add seasonings. Add cooked spinach, cheese and reheat. Stuff both manicotti with vegetable mixture and put in a baking dish. Top each manicotti with salmon sauce. Cover and bake at 350 °F/180 °C for 15 minutes. Makes 2 servings.

Salmon (canned)	4 oz (120 g)
Cream soup (celery) (low fat)	¼ cup (60 ml)
Plain yogurt, 2 %	2 tbsp (30 ml)
Parsley, chopped	1 tbsp (15 ml)
Manicotti, cooked	2
Garlic clove, crushed	1
Shallot, chopped	1 tbsp (15 ml)
Basil	¼ tsp (1 ml)
Spinach, chopped and cooked	¼ cup (60 ml)
Cottage Cheese, 1 %	½ cup (125 ml)
Salt and black pepper, to taste	

For one serving:

Carbohydrates:	20 g = 5 units
Fat:	5 g = 1 unit
Proteins:	24 g
Calories:	230

❖

Spaghetti

First combine meat, onion powder and pepper. Then shape into meatballs (6). Broil them at 350 °F/180 °C for 15 minutes. In a casserole, cook bean sprouts on medium heat for 15 minutes. Combine the remaining ingredients and prepare sauce. On medium heat, cook green pepper until tender, about 15 minutes. When sauce is ready add meatballs and cook 5 minutes more. Serve sauce on bean sprouts. Makes 2 servings.

Beef, lean ground	7 oz (210 g)
Bean sprouts	2 cups (500 ml)
Tomato juice	½ cup (125 ml)
Tomatoes, sliced	2 small
Green pepper, chopped	¼ cup (60 ml)
Shallot, chopped	2 tbsp (30 ml)
Onion powder	½ tsp (2 ml)
Basil, fresh	3 leaves
Oregano	¼ tsp (1 ml)
Salt	½ tsp (2 ml)

For one serving:

Carbohydrates:	17 g	= 4 units
Fat:	14 g	= 3 units
Proteins:	23 g	
Calories:	278	

❖

Cheese Bows

Place cooked pasta and cubed carrots in a greased baking dish. Combine cottage cheese with milk and salt; whisk with electric beater. Spread cheese mixture over pasta and carrots. Cover and bake at 350 °F/180 °C for 10 minutes.

TOPPING:

Mix shallots with garlic, basil, parsley, bread crumbs and parmesan cheese. Pour topping over pasta and broil for 2 minutes. Makes 2 servings.

Bows, (pasta) cooked	1 ½ cup (375 ml)
Carrot, cubed and cooked	½ cup (125 ml)
Cottage Cheese	1 cup (250 ml)
2 % partially skimmed milk	2 tbsp (30 ml)
Salt, to taste	

TOPPING:	
Shallot, chopped	1 tbsp (15 ml)
Garlic clove, chopped	1
Basil	3 leaves
Parsley, chopped (fresh)	1 tsp (5 ml)
Bread crumbs	1 tsp (5 ml)
Parmesan cheese, grated	1 tbsp (15 ml)

For one serving:
Carbohydrates: 60 g = 15 units
Fat: 5 g = 1 unit
Proteins: 27 g
Calories: 400

❖

Scrambled Eggs with Shallot

Beat the eggs and add skim milk, shallots, salt and pepper; mix well. Pour into a non-stick pan and cook on medium heat. Stir. Remove eggs from heat while they are still soft. Put in a serving dish and garnish with chopped parsley. Serve. Makes 1 serving.

Eggs (medium)	2
Skimmed milk	2 tbsp (30 ml)
Shallot, chopped	2 tbsp (30 ml)
Salt, black pepper and parsley, to taste	

For one serving:

Carbohydrates:	3 g = 1 unit
Fat:	11 g = 2 units
Proteins:	13 g
Calories:	164

❖

Scrambled Eggs and Vegetables

Beat eggs with a fork. Add water and salt. Mix well. Heat a frying pan (without oil or butter) and cook onion, zucchini and green pepper over medium heat. Add eggs. Using a wooden spatula, stir. Remove eggs from heat while they are still soft. Makes 1 serving.

Eggs	2
Onion, chopped	2 tsp (10 ml)
Water	2 tbsp (30 ml)
Zucchini, cubed	½ cup (125 ml)
Green pepper, cubed	½ cup (125 ml)
Salt	¼ tsp (1 ml)

For one serving:

Carbohydrates:	13 g = 3 units
Fat:	10 g = 2 units
Proteins:	15 g
Calories:	201

Egg Florentine

In a casserole, combine water and vinegar. Microwave at full power for 2 minutes or until boiling. Break egg into the casserole with water and vinegar. Prick egg yolk. Cover and microwave at full power for 1 ½ minute. Wash spinach and discard stems. Microwave at full power for 2 minutes. Drain well and chop spinach coarsely. Spoon spinach onto serving dish and place egg over spinach. Spoon yogurt over egg and sprinkle grated cheese. Microwave at full power for 20 to 30 seconds. Makes 1 serving.

Egg	1
Spinach	1 cup (250 ml)
Plain yogurt	1 tbsp (15 ml)
Low fat cheese, grated	1 tbsp (15 ml)
Water	3 cups (750 ml)
Vinegar (optional)	½ tsp (2 ml)

For one serving:
Carbohydrates: 3 g = 1 unit
Fat: 8 g = 1.5 units
Proteins: 12 g
Calories: 133

Poached Eggs with Tomatoes

In a non-stick pan, cook the onion on medium heat until tender and add garlic and cook for 30 seconds. Combine tomatoes with seasonings and simmer over low heat until tomato mixture thickens slightly. Break eggs into a small bowl. Make 2 holes in the tomato mixture and gently drop each egg into the mixture. Cover and cook eggs on low heat for 3 to 4 minutes until whites are firm. Serve on warm rice. Makes 1 serving.

Eggs	2
Onion, chopped	¼ cup (60 ml)
Garlic clove, crushed	1
Tomatoes (canned)	1 cup (250 ml)
Oregano	¼ tsp (1 ml)
Rice (long grains), cooked	½ cup (125 ml)
Salt and black pepper	1 pinch

For one serving:

Carbohydrates:	41 g = 8 units
Fat:	12 g = 2.5 units
Proteins:	18 g
Calories:	339

❖

Omelet with Ham and Zucchini

In a bowl, beat eggs with water and seasoning. In a non-stick pan, cook onions until tender. Add zucchini and cook for 5 minutes until tender. Add meat and cook on medium heat for 2 minutes. Stir. Pour beaten eggs over cooked zucchini. Stir rapidly. Sprinkle with grated cheese. Place omelet in oven and bake it until it becomes brown and rises. Makes 2 servings.

Eggs	2
Water	2 tbsp (30 ml)
Onion, chopped	¼ cup (60 ml)
Zucchini, thinly sliced	½ cup (125 ml)
Ham, ground (cooked)	1 oz (30 g)
Mozzarella skimmed cheese, grated	1 oz (30 g)
Salt and black pepper, to taste	

For one serving:

Carbohydrates:	5 g = 1 unit
Fat:	9 g = 2 units
Proteins:	14 g
Calories:	162

❖

Spanish Omelet

Cover and microwave all vegetables, except tomato, at full power for 1 ½ minute. In bowl, mix eggs, pepper, oregano and salt. Microwave the mixture at full power for 40 seconds. Place vegetables on the omelet and fold it. Microwave at full power for 50 seconds. Garnish with parsley and serve. Makes 1 serving.

Eggs (beaten)	2
Fresh celery, diced	¼ cup (60 ml)
Green pepper, cubed	½ cup (125 ml)
Tomatoes, wedges	4
Oregano	½ tsp (2 ml)
Parsley	1 bouquet
Salt and black pepper, to taste	

For one serving:

Carbohydrates: 16 g = 4 units
Fat: 11 g = 2 units
Proteins: 15
Calories: 217

Basil Omelet

Mix all the ingredients together. Beat lightly. Pour into a non-stick skillet and cook over low heat. With a spatula, lift the omelet to permit the liquid to reach the bottom of the pan. Cook until golden. Fold the omelets in two. Makes 1 serving.

Eggs (medium)	2
Water	2 tbsp (30 ml)
Basil, fresh	¼ tsp (1 ml)
Parsley, chopped	¼ tsp (1 ml)
Salt	1 pinch
Black pepper, to taste	

For one serving:
Carbohydrates: 2 g = 0.5 unit
Fat: 10 g = 2 units
Proteins: 13 g
Calories: 149

❖

Mushroom and Cheese Omelet

Combine all ingredients and beat slightly. Pour egg mixture into a non-stick pan. Cook on low heat until omelet has browned. Garnish with parsley before serving. Makes 1 serving.

Eggs	2
Water	1 tsp (5 ml)
Low fat cheese, grated	1 oz (30 g)
Fresh mushrooms, sliced	2 tbsp (30 ml)
Onion, chopped	1 tbsp (15 ml)
Salt, black pepper and parsley, to taste	

For one serving:
Carbohydrates: 4 g = 1 unit
Fat: 11 g = 2 units
Proteins: 15 g
Calories: 175

Mushroom/Asparagus Omelet

Mix all ingredients. Beat lightly. Pour the mixture into a non-stick skillet, heated slightly. Cook slowly at low heat. With a spatula lift the omelet as to let the liquid spread to the bottom of the skillet. Cook until the bottom of the omelet is done. Slip the omelets into a plate and fold. Serve. Makes 1 serving.

Eggs	2
Water	2 tbsp (30 ml)
Shallot, chopped finely	1 tsp (5 ml)
Fresh mushrooms, sliced	2 tbsp (30 ml)
Asparagus tips	2 tbsp (30 ml)
Tarragon	1 pinch
Parsley, to taste	
Salt, to taste	
Black pepper, to taste	

For one serving:

Carbohydrates:	3 g	= 1 unit
Fat:	10 g	= 2 units
Proteins:	14 g	
Calories:	163	

❖

Omelet with Zucchini

Peel zucchini and cut into cubes. Place zucchini in baking dish and add tomato sauce and garlic. Microwave, covered, at full power for 1 minute. In bowl beat eggs, add salt, pepper, parsley and cubed zucchini. Place mixture in baking dish and microwave at full power for 2 minutes. Garnish with parsley and serve. Makes 1 serving.

Eggs	2
Tomato sauce	1 tbsp (15 ml)
Zucchini	½ cup (125 ml)
Garlic clove, chopped	½
Parsley, chopped	1 tsp (5 ml)
Salt and black pepper, to taste	

For one serving:
Carbohydrates: 7 g = 2 units
Fat:　　　　　 10 g = 2 units
Proteins:　　　 14 g
Calories:　　　 174

❖

Fine Herbs Omelet

In a bowl, beat eggs and add fine herbs, a little salt and pepper. Microwave, uncovered, at full power for 1 ½ minute. Garnish with parsley and serve. Makes 1 serving.

Eggs	2
Chives	½ tsp (2 ml)
Fine herbs	½ tsp (2 ml)
Salt, black pepper and parsley, to taste	

For one serving:
Carbohydrates: 1 g
Fat:　　　　　 10 g = 2 units
Proteins:　　　 13 g
Calories:　　　 150

Herb Omelet

Beat egg whites until stiff. Beat yolks with water and herbs and spices. Fold into whites. Cook in a non-stick skillet until set. Top with cheese and transfer to 350 °F/180 °C oven, bake 2 minutes. Makes 1 serving.

Eggs (separated)	2
Water	2 tbsp (30 ml)
Parsley	½ tsp (2 ml)
Chives	½ tsp (2 ml)
Marjoram	1 pinch
Thyme	1 pinch
Cheese	2 oz (60 g)
Tarragon	1 pinch
Mozarella skimmed cheese grated	2 oz (60 g)
Salt and black pepper, to taste	

For one serving:

Carbohydrates:	2 g = 0.5 unit
Fat:	24 g = 5 units
Proteins:	26 g
Calories:	375

❖

Spanish Omelet

Scramble the eggs with the butter. Add the mushrooms, tomatoes and green pepper. Simmer for 5 minutes, stir and top with cheese. Cover and simmer 5 to 10 minutes longer or until cheese melts. Makes 1 serving.

Eggs, beaten	2
Fresh mushrooms, sliced	¼ cup (60 ml)
Tomato, chopped	½
Green pepper, chopped	¼ cup (60 ml)
Mozarella skimmed cheese, grated	2 oz (60 g)
Butter	2 tsp (10 ml)

For one serving:
Carbohydrates: 9 g = 2 units
Fat: 28 g = 5.5 units
Proteins: 28 g
Calories: 395

❖

Spring Omelet

In a bowl, combine eggs with cheese, mushrooms, cubed asparagus stems (keep asparagus tips as garnish) and tarragon. Add pepper and a little salt. Place the ingredients in microwave dish and microwave, covered, at full power for 2 minutes. Garnish with asparagus tips and serve. Makes 1 serving.

Eggs	2
Cottage Cheese	2 tbsp (30 ml)
Fresh mushrooms, minced	2
Asparagus stalks	4
Tarragon	¼ tsp (1 ml)
Salt and black pepper, to taste	

For one serving:

Carbohydrates:	6 g = 1.5 units
Fat:	11 g = 2 units
Proteins:	18 g
Calories:	191

❖

Turkey Quiche

Beat eggs lightly and add other ingredients. Pour into an 8-inch (20 cm) quiche dish (sprayed with Pam) and cook at 350 °F (180 °C) for 30 minutes. Cut into six slices. Makes 6 servings.

Eggs, beaten	10
Green pepper, chopped	2
Parsley	2 tsp (10 ml)
Oregano	1 tsp (5 ml)
Turkey or chicken, cooked, diced	2 cups (500 ml)
Onion, chopped	2 tbsp (30 ml)
Chili flakes	2 tsp (10 ml)
Clove garlic, chopped	1
Salt and black pepper, to taste	

For one serving:

Carbohydrates:	3 g = 1 unit
Fat:	13 g = 2.5 units
Proteins:	21 g
Calories:	222

❖

Broccoli and Cheese Quiche

Cook broccoli. Beat eggs and add chicken broth dissolved in water. Beat again. Put broccoli in a casserole sprayed with Pam. Sprinkle with shredded cheese and then pour egg mixture (beaten well) over broccoli and cheese. Season to taste. Bake at 350 °F/ 180 °C until top is brown. Makes 3 servings.

Broccoli, cooked	2 cups (500 ml)
Water	½ cup (125 ml)
Chicken broth, fat free	1 pouch
Cheddar cheese (mild)	8 oz (240 g)
Eggs	4
Chives, chopped	2 tsp (10 ml)
Salt	1 tsp (5 ml)
Black pepper	1 tsp (5 ml)

For one serving:

Carbohydrates:	12 g = 3 units
Fat:	32 g = 6.5 units
Proteins:	33 g
Calories:	457

❖

Asparagus Quiche

Heat oven to 375 °F/190 °C. In a small saucepan, cook shallots until tender. In bowl, combine them with milk, asparagus, eggs and half of the grated cheese. Season and mix well. Grease quiche dish with butter and pour in the egg mixture. Sprinkle with the remaining grated cheese. Bake at 375 °F/ 190 °C for 35 minutes. Makes 2 servings.

Butter	1 tsp (5 ml)
Shallot, chopped	¼ cup (60 ml)
Asparagus, cooked	1 cup (250 ml)
Skimmed milk	½ cup (125 ml)
Eggs, beaten	2
Gruyère cheese, grated	2 oz (60 g)
Cayenne pepper	1 pinch
Salt	1 pinch
Black pepper	¼ tsp (1 ml)

For one serving:

Carbohydrates:	10 g = 2.5 units
Fat:	18 g = 3.5 units
Proteins:	20 g
Calories:	274

❖

Vegetables Quiche, traditional oven

Lightly sauté garlic, onions, vegetables. Meanwhile, mix eggs, cheese and seasonings. Mix into vegetables and pour into a lightly oiled casserole. Bake at 350 °F/180 °C for 30 minutes. Makes 3 servings.

Broccoli, cauliflower and squash	3 cups (750 ml)
Onion minced	¼ cup (60 ml)
Garlic clove, minced	3
Eggs	6
Cheese, grated	6 oz (180 g)
Thyme	1 tsp (5 ml)
Basil	1 tsp (5 ml)
Garlic powder	2 tsp (10 ml)
Water	3 tsp (15 ml)

For one serving:

Carbohydrates:	20 g = 5 units
Fat:	15 g = 3 units
Proteins:	36 g
Calories:	339

❖

Vegetables Quiche, microwave

In a microwave-safe dish, place washed broccoli and cauliflower. Microwave at full power for 2 minutes. In a small bowl, mix eggs with cheese, onion and paprika. Add salt and pepper. Place all vegetables in quiche dish and pour egg mixture over the vegetables. Microwave, uncovered, at full power for 2 minutes. Makes 1 serving.

Eggs	2
Gruyère cheese, grated	1 oz (30 g)
Broccoli	½ cup (125 ml)
Cauliflower	½ cup (125 ml)
Fresh mushrooms, minced	3
Onion, chopped	1 tbsp (15 ml)
Paprika, to taste	
Salt, to taste	
Black pepper, to taste	

For one serving:

Carbohydrates:	16 g = 4 units
Fat:	20 g = 5 units
Proteins:	29 g
Calories:	335

❖

Seafood Quiche

Put spinach leaves in microwave-safe dish and microwave at full power for 1 minute. Chill, drain and put in a small quiche dish. Microwave shrimp and crab at fully power for 30 seconds. Add all other ingredients, except cheese. Microwave at medium-high (70 %) for 2 minutes. Makes 1 serving.

Canned crab, minced	1 oz (30 g)
Shrimp, minced	1 oz (30 g)
Onion, chopped	1 tsp (5 ml)
Skimmed milk	1 tbsp (15 ml)
Mozzarella skimmed cheese, part. skimmed	1 tbsp (15 ml)
Egg	1
Paprika	1 pinch
Spinach	6 leaves
Salt, to taste	
Black pepper, to taste	

For one serving:
Carbohydrates: 3 g = 1 unit
Fat: 9 g = 2 units
Proteins: 23 g
Calories: 192

❖

Traditional Quiche

Beat eggs lightly and stir in other ingredients. Pour into a small
quiche dish (sprayed with Pam) and cook at 350 °F (180 °C) for
15 to 20 minutes. Serve hot. Makes 2 servings.

Eggs, beaten	3
Green pepper, chopped	½ cup (125 ml)
Parsley, chopped	½ cup (2 ml)
Oregano	1 pinch
Chicken, cooked, diced	¾ cup (180 ml)
Onion, chopped	2 tsp (10 ml)
Clove garlic, sliced	1
Salt and black pepper	

For one serving:
Carbohydrates: 4 g = 1 unit
Fat: 12 g = 2.5 units
Proteins: 17 g
Calories: 190

❖

Chocolate Drink

Mix in blender and enjoy. Makes 1 serving.

Water (cold)	1 cup (250 ml)
Chocolate milk skimmed	1 cup (250 ml)
Cottage Cheese	1 tbsp (15 ml)
Water (ice cubes)	3
Sugar substitute	1 envelope

For one serving:
Carbohydrates: 28 g = 7 units
Fat: 5 g = 1 unit
Proteins: 11 g
Calories: 203

Strawberry Shake

Soften the gelatin in cold water. Add the hot water to fully dissolve the gelatin. Add strawberries, vanilla, sugar and salt; mix well. Refrigerate until the mixture has partially hardened. Beat the mixture until it is thick and foamy. Beat the egg whites, add to the mixture and continue to beat until it is firm. Pour into 6 dessert cups (½ cup each). Cool. Garnish each cup with half a strawberry. Makes 6 servings.

Gelatin (unflavored)	1 pouch
Water (cold)	¼ cup (60 ml)
Water (hot)	¼ cup (60 ml)
Fresh strawberries or frozen	2 cups (500 ml)
Vanilla	½ tsp (2 ml)
Sugar substitute	½ tsp (2 ml)
Egg whites	2
Salt	¼ tsp (1 ml)

For one serving:

Carbohydrates:	3 g = 1 unit
Fat:	1 g
Proteins:	2 g
Calories:	26

❖

Poached Apples

Carefully mix all the ingredients in a casserole. Cook at very low heat, covered for about 30 minutes. This can be served hot or cold. Makes 1 serving.

Apples (red), sliced	1 ½ cup (375 ml)
Orange juice, unsweetened	¼ cup (60 ml)
Cinnamon	¼ tsp (1 ml)
Sugar substitute	1 pouch

For one serving:
Carbohydrates: 56 g = 14 units
Fat: 1 g
Proteins: 1 g
Calories: 216

❖

Fruit Salad

Mix all ingredients and put in the refrigerator. Makes 3 servings.

Apple, in pieces	1
Grapes, green	½ cup (125 ml)
Banana, sliced	½
Raisins	1 tbsp (15 ml)
Plain yogurt, 2 %	3 tbsp (45 ml)

For one serving:
Carbohydrates: 21 g = 5 units
Fat: 2 g = 0.5 unit
Proteins: 1 g
Calories: 101

Fresh Fruit Salad

Peel, remove pit and cut up peach. Cut strawberries in two. Remove the membrane on the grapefruit. Cut it up. Remove the core leaving, the skin on the apple. Add to strawberries and peach. Add lemon juice to prevent fruit from darkening. Add vanilla and sugar. Let stand for a few hours in the fridge. Makes 4 servings.

Peach	1
Fresh strawberries	½ cup (125 ml)
Apple, green or red	1
Grapefruit, in quarters	½
Lemon juice	¼ tsp (1 ml)
Sugar substitute	¼ tsp (1 ml)
Vanilla	¼ tsp (1 ml)

For one serving:

Carbohydrates:	12 g = 3 units
Fat:	Trace amount
Proteins:	Trace amount
Calories:	50

❖

Fish or Chicken Aspic

Sprinkle the gelatin in cold water. Allow the gelatin to dissolve over the hot water of a double boiler. Add lemon and seasoning. When the gelatin begins to solidify, add the fish or chicken and celery. Fold in mayonnaise, put in refrigerator and serve with cucumber vinaigrette. Makes 4 servings.

Gelatin, plain	1 envelope
Water	¼ cup (60 ml)
Lemon juice	2 tbsp (30 ml)
Dry mustard	1 tsp (5 ml)
Paprika	¼ tsp (1 ml)
Tuna, crabmeat or cooked chicken	2 cups (500 ml)
Celery, chopped	1 cup (250 ml)
Mayonnaise, light	¼ cup (60 ml)
Salt, to taste	

For one serving:

Carbohydrates:	3 g = 1 unit
Fat:	8 g = 1.5 units
Proteins:	26 g
Calories:	188

❖

Chicken Aspic

Sprinkle the gelatin in ½ cup (125 ml) of the chicken broth. Mix over low heat to dissolve the gelatin, add the rest of the broth. Refrigerate to allow gelatin to solidify. Add the rest of the ingredients to the broth and demold on a 9" x 5" x 3" (23 cm x 13 cm x 8 cm) plate. Allow to cool. Makes 4 servings.

Gelatin, plain	1 envelope
Chicken broth, fat free	1 cup (250 ml)
Cooked chicken, diced	2 cups (500 ml)
Lemon juice	2 tbsp (30 ml)
Celery, chopped	¼ cup (60 ml)
Onion, sliced	1 tbsp (15 ml)
Parsley	1 tsp (5 ml)
Salt, to taste	

For one serving:

Carbohydrates:	2 g	= 0.5 unit
Fat:	14 g	= 3 units
Proteins:	27 g	
Calories:	251	

❖

Vegetable Aspic

Dilute the gelatin in hot water. Add salt, vinegar, lemon and pour half of the gelatin into a dish. Put in the refrigerator until the gelatin starts to solidify. While the gelatin is in the refrigerator, cook the beans in the boiling water in a pot, and the rest of the vegetables in another pot. Put cooked beans in the chilled gelatin. Mix the rest of the gelatin with the other cooked vegetables and pour this mixture over the first mixture. Demold and cut into squares. Makes 4 servings.

Gelatin, plain	2 envelopes
Boiling water	3 ½ cup (875 ml)
Vinegar, white (optional)	1 tbsp (15 ml)
Lemon juice (optional)	1 tbsp (15 ml)
Green beans	2 ½ cups (625 ml)
Cauliflower, in pieces	½
Broccoli, in pieces	½
Celery, chopped	½ cup (125 ml)
Radishes	6
Salt, to taste (optional)	

For one serving:
Carbohydrates: 14 g = 3.5 units
Fat: 1 g
Proteins: 8 g
Calories: 87

❖

Cheese Patties

In a bowl, combine all ingredients. Mix well and shape into 4 patties. Then, place on a baking sheet sprayed with Pam. Bake at 375 °F/190 °C for 10 minutes. Makes 2 servings.

Skimmed Cottage Cheese	½ cup (125 ml)
Low fat cheddar cheese, grated	½ cup (125 ml)
Gruyère cheese, grated	½ cup (125 ml)
Bread crumbs	⅓ cup (80 ml)
Parsley, chopped (fresh)	1 tbsp (15 ml)
Shallot, chopped	2
Basil	1 pinch
Egg	1 (beaten)
Mustard, powder	1 pinch

For one serving:

Carbohydrates:	18 g = 4.5 units
Fat:	26 g = 5 units
Proteins:	46 g
Calories:	502

❖

Jambalaya

Cook the brown rice in chicken broth (about 20 minutes). Meanwhile, brown onion and green peas on medium heat for 3 minutes. Add tomatoes, garlic, thyme, pepper, ham and cooked rice. Mix well. Finally, top with cooked shrimp and sprinkle with parsley. Cover and bake at 350 °F/180 °C for 10 minutes. Makes 2 servings.

Rice (uncooked brown)	¼ cup (60 ml)
Chicken broth, fat free	½ cup (125 ml)
Onion, chopped	¼ cup (60 ml)
Peas, frozen	¼ cup (60 ml)
Tomatoes, chopped	1 cup (250 ml)
Garlic clove, chopped	1
Thyme	¼ tsp (1 ml)
Ham strips	4 oz (120 g)
Shrimp, frozen (cooked)	2 oz (60 g)
Parsley (fresh), chopped	1 tsp (5 ml)
Black pepper	¼ tsp (1 ml)

For one serving:
Carbohydrates: 34 g = 8.5 units
Fat: 4 g = 1 unit
Proteins: 22 g
Calories: 255

❖

Moussaka

In a non-stick pan, brown the beef on medium heat. Add vegetables and seasonings. Cook on medium heat for 5 minutes.

SAUCE:

Heat milk and onions until to a boils. Add cornstarch dissolved in cold water. Season and cook until mixture thickens (stirring). Spread bread crumbs at the bottom of a baking dish. Place half the quantity of eggplant mixture, add half the quantity of sauce and alternate. Pour the beaten egg over and garnish with grated cheese. Bake at 350 °F/180 °C for 40 minutes. Makes 2 servings.

Beef, lean ground	6 oz (180 g)
Eggplant, peeled and sliced	1 small
Onion, sliced	½ cup (125 ml)
Tomatoes	½ cup (125 ml)
Parsley (fresh), chopped	1 tbsp (15 ml)
Salt, black pepper and oregano, to taste	

SAUCE:

2 % partially skimmed milk	1 cup (250 ml)
Low fat mozzarella cheese, grated	¼ cup (60 ml)
Cornstarch	1 tbsp (15 ml)
Water (cold)	2 tbsp (30 ml)
Bread crumbs	2 tbsp (30 ml)
Eggs (beaten)	1

For one serving:

Carbohydrates:	56 g = 9 units
Fat:	26 g = 5 units
Proteins:	40 g
Calories:	622

❖

English Muffin with Tuna

Place the English muffin in a microwave-safe dish and garnish with onion slice. Combine all ingredients except the cheese. Spread mixture on muffin and top it with the cheese. Microwave at medium-high for 1 or 2 minutes until cheese has melted. Serve. Makes 1 serving.

English muffin, grilled	½
Onion	1 slice
Tuna (canned)	2 oz (60 g)
Mayonnaise, light	1 tsp (5 ml)
Dijon mustard	¼ tsp (1 ml)
Celery seeds	¼ tsp (1 ml)
Cheddar cheese, 7 %, grated	½ oz (15 g)
Alfalfa	

For one serving:

Carbohydrates:	16 g = 4 units
Fat:	6 g = 1 unit
Proteins:	23 g
Calories:	21

❖

Welsh Rarebit-Ham Sandwich

Place slice of ham on bread and top with slice of cheese. Garnish with green pepper slice. Broil at 475 °F/250 °C until cheese melts. Makes 1 serving.

Sliced bread, toasted   1 slice
Ham (cooked)   2 oz (60 g)
Gruyère cheese   2 tbsp (30 ml)
Green pepper   1 slice
Mustard   1 tsp (5 ml)

For one serving:
Carbohydrates: 14 g = 3.5 units
Fat: 13 g = 2.5 units
Proteins: 22 g
Calories: 261

❖

Index Recipes

– A –

Almond Chicken, 150
Alsatian Sole, 190
Asparagus Chicken, 126
Asparagus Quiche, 274
Asparagus Tips, 240

– B –

Baked Mixed Vegetables, 232
Baked Salmon, 185
Baked Salmon with Curry, 171
Baked Sole, 191
Baked Stuffed Mushrooms Florentine, 215
Basil Omelet, 266
Bean Sprouts with Italian Rice, 222
Bean Sprouts, Alfalfa and Spinach, 223
Beef and Carrots, 74
Beef and Tomato Stew, 87
Beef and Vegetables, microwave, 77
Beef Brochette, 84
Beef Cannelloni, 256
Beef Chow Mein, 89
Beef Sandwich, 92
Beef Strips, 96

Beef Stroganov, 81
Beef with Vegetables, traditional oven, 76
Bitter-Sweet Pork and Pineapple, 105
Bouillabaisse Gaspésienne, 168
Braised Beef with Carrots, 79
Braised Veal with Mushrooms, 125
Broccoli and Cheese Quiche, 273
Broccoli or Cauliflower in Tomato Sauce, 217
Broiled Tomato, 226

– C –

Calf's Liver with Basil, 99
Calf's Liver with Green Pepper, 103
Calf's Liver with Vegetable, 102
Calf's Liver with White Leek, 100
Cantonese Beef, 72
Cantonese Chicken, 134
Caraway Cabbage, 218
Cauliflower and Artichoke, 219
Ceasar Salad, 247
Cheese Bows, 260
Cheese Dip, 236
Cheese Patties, 285
Chicken à l'Orange, 131

Chicken à la Crème, 135
Chicken à la Mode, 136
Chicken Alexandra, 141
Chicken and Egg Salad, 252
Chicken Ascar, 143
Chicken Aspic, 283
Chicken Basquaise, 157
Chicken Brunswick, 158
Chicken Chop Suey, 130
Chicken Dijon, 137
Chicken Gumbo, 160
Chicken Jardinière, 161
Chicken and Vegetables, 162
Chicken Liver Brochette, 97
Chicken Livers, 98
Chicken Maria, 163
Chicken or Turkey Salad, 245
Chicken Provençal, 138
Chicken Rice with Fruit, 164
Chicken Salad, 251
Chicken Steak, 165
Chicken with Apple, 155
Chicken with Broccoli, 144
Chicken with Curry, 145
Chicken with Fine Herbs, 151
Chicken with Fresh Peach, 154
Chicken with Green Pepper, 148
Chicken with Orange, 142
Chicken with Peaches, 153
Chicken Zucchini Salad, 251
Chinese Beef with Tomatoes, 78
Chinese Meatballs, 83
Chocolate Drink, 278
Chop Suey, 88
Cod Bergeronne, 182
Cod with Vegetables, 181
Confetti Salad, 252
Coq au Vin, 132
Coquille Saint-Jacques, microwave,
175
Coquille St-Jacques, traditional oven,
174
Country Casserole, 71
Crab Salad, 242
Cream and Mushrooms Beef, 73
Cucumber Salad, 240

– D –
Deviled Chicken Legs, 133
Dilled Zucchini, 203
Doria Sole, 195

– E –
Egg and Cottage Salad, 238
Eggs and Vegetables Salad, 236
Egg Florentine, 262
Eggplant Marinade, 203
English Muffin with Tuna, 288

– F –
Fillet of Sole Dieppoise, 193
Fine Herbs Omelet, 268
Fine Herbs Patty, 79
Fish Casserole with Tomato, 172
Fish Créole, 188
Fish Fillet à la Créole, 187
Fish Fillet Provençal, 189
Fish Fillet with Orange, 189
Fish or Chicken Aspic, 282
Fisherman's Chowder, 173
Fresh Fruit Salad, 281
Fruit Salad, 280

– G –
Garden Vegetable Casserole, 231
Gazpacho, 229
Ginger Chicken with Peaches, 147
Goulash, 93
Green Bean and Sprout Salad, 249
Green Pepper Steak, 68

– H –

Haddock Bonne-Femme, 167
Haddock with Celery, 166
Halibut with Lemon, 179
Halibut with Vegetables, 178
Ham Rolls, 109
Hawaiian Salad, 253
Herb Omelet, 269
Hot Crab Salad, 243
Hot Salmon and Cabbage Salad, 239
Hot Spinach Salad, 246
Hungarian Veal Cutlets, 117

– I –

Indian Meatballs, 112
Indian Veal, 122
Isabelle Steak, 69
Italian Beef Cubes, 91
Italian Meat Loaf, 94
Italian Steak, 66

– J –

Jambalaya, 286

– L –

Lamb Brochettes, 64
Lamb Loaf, 65
Lamb with Orange, 63
Legume Loaf, 233
Lemon Chicken, 146
Liver with Fine Herbs, 101

– M –

Macaroni with Beef au Gratin, 257
Mandarin Chicken, 152
Manicotti with Salmon Sauce, 258
Meatball Brochettes, 85
Meatballs with Green Pepper, 86
Milanese Stuffed Zucchini, 208
Mock Sour Cream Dip, 235
Molded Garden Relish, 230

Moussaka, 287
Mushroom and Cheese Omelet, 266
Mushroom Delight, 216
Mushroom/Asparagus Omelet, 267
Mushroom Snacks, 214

– O –

Omelet with Ham and Zucchini, 264
Omelet with Zucchini, 268
Oriental Steak, 67
Oriental Turkey Casserole, 130

– P –

Paprika Veal Cutlet, 118
Parisian Patties, 90
Peking Calf's Liver, 102
Pepper Steak, 68
Perfection Salad, 254
Pescado à la Naranja (halibut), 184
Pineapple Pork, 106
Poached Apples, 280
Poached Cod and Mushroom Sauce, 183
Poached Eggs with Tomatoes, 263
Pork "Fried" Rice, 108
Pork Meatballs with Tomatoes, 104
Pork with Onion and Apples, 107
Portuguese Cod Fillet, 180
Pressure Cooked Chicken, 149
Provençal Tuna (1), 199
Provençal Tuna (2), 200

– R –

Ratatouille Niçoise, 234
Rice Loaf with Carrot, 232
Roasted Peppers, 212
Rolled Boston Bluefish, 177

– S –

Salmon Steak with Dill, 176
Salmon with Shrimp, 186

Sauted Chicken Livers, 99
Scrambled Eggs and Vegetables, 261
Scrambled Eggs with Shallot, 261
Seafood Brochette (1), 169
Seafood Brochette (2), 170
Seafood Quiche, 277
Seasoned Meat Loaf, 95
Sole Dijonnaise, 194
Sole Fillet en Verdure, 196
Sole Fillet Gratiné, 197
Sole Fillet Marinière, 198
Sole Niçoise, 198
Sole with Clams, 192
Soup Supreme, 235
Spaghetti, 259
Spanish Chicken, 139
Spanish Omelet, 265, 270
Spiced Pear Salad, 237
Spicy Veal Cutlet, 120
Spinach and Lemon, 212
Spinach Casserole, 213
Spinach Gourmet, 213
Spinach Soufflé, 214
Spinach-Sprout Salad, 248
Spring Omelet, 271
Spring Salad, 255
Squash Bake, 204
Stir-fried Cabbage, 221
Stir-Fry, 228
Strawberry Shake, 279
Stuffed Cabbage, 219
Stuffed Chicken, 160
Stuffed Cucumber, 227
Stuffed Eggplant, 202
Stuffed Green Pepper, 211
Stuffed Pepper with Cheese, 210
Stuffed Pepper, traditional oven, 209
Stuffed Zucchini (1), 206
Stuffed Zucchini (2), 207
Super Tomatoes, 226

Surprise Ground Steak, 80
Swedish Meatballs, 82
Sweet–and–Sour Pork and Pineapple, 105
Swiss Steak, 70

– T –

Tangy Green Beans, 223
Tangy Mustard Beans, 224
Tangy Wilted Spinach Salad, 250
Tangy Zucchini, 205
Tarragon Chicken, 140
Tarragon Patty, 86
Tasty Green Beans, 224
Tasty Red Cabbage, 220
Tasty Shrimp Salad, 244
Teriyaki Chicken Brochette, 128
Tomato Turkey Meatballs, 127
Traditional Quiche, 278
Tuna Cucumber Boats, 201
Tuna-Stuffed Tomato, 225
Turkey Casserole, 129
Turkey Quiche, 272
Turkey Roast with Fine Herbs, 165

– V –

Veal Blanquette, 111
Veal Brochette, 113
Veal Croquette, 116
Veal Cutlet au Gratin, 118
Veal Cutlet Bonne-Femme, 115
Veal Cutlet Parmesan, 119
Veal Meatballs with Chervil, 114
Veal Patties, 121
Veal Steak with Paprika, 110
Veal with Carrots, 123
Veal with Fine Herbs, 124
Vegetable Aspic, 284
Vegetables and Beef, 75
Vegetables Quiche, microwave, 276

Vegetables Quiche, traditional oven,
275
Vinegar Chicken, 140

– W –

Welsh Rarebit-Ham Sandwich, 289
Wild Chicken, 159

– Y –

Yogurt and Mushroom Chicken, 156

– Z –

Zucchini Slaw, 241